WIRED TO BE DYSFUNCTIONAL

Wired to be Dysfunctional

OUR JOURNEY WITH MYOCLONUS DYSTONIA

Brianna Lafferty

Jill Lafferty

BriOnic LLC

Contents

Medical Disclaimer

The content of this book is not intended to be a substitute for professional medical advice, diagnosis, or treatment of any physical, emotional, or medical condition. Always seek the medical advice of your physician or other qualified medical professionals regarding any medical condition. The content of this book is for informational purposes only. Should you decide to forgo appropriate professional medical advice and rely on any information provided in this book for self-treatment, you do so at your own risk. The authors and the publisher of this book assume no liability for your actions.

The names of the people referred to in this book have been given initials, in order to protect their identities.

Prologue

From a very young age, I had envisioned being a fantastic and fun-loving youthful mom. I dreamt about all of the exciting things I would do with my babies, and how my babies would respond to me and my nurturing. I had a ton of love to give, and I knew that I would be a natural at being a mom. I had visions of cherubic babies nursing with ease getting chubby, sleeping well, reaching milestones on time, and absolutely thriving. My babies would be very happy and content. Boy, was I in for a rude awakening. Except for an easy and uneventful pregnancy, with a four-hour delivery using self-hypnosis, my idyllic vision of motherhood would soon be shattered. The majority of the next 31 years with my beautiful baby girl, Bri, would be very challenging, sometimes excruciatingly so; yet bittersweet with the realization that we are all much stronger and more resilient than we realize. This is our story of letting expectations go; of living life not according to plan; of becoming resilient; and of finding hope and happiness in the journey. We hope this journey of discovery inspires you to be the best advocate, for yourself or for your loved one. Never give up; there is always hope and you may have to fight for it. When the answers start to align and make sense, the battle will have been worth the effort.

1

A Mama's Perspective

On September 24, 1991, I realized my dream of becoming a mother with the birth of my first child, Brianna Nicole. We chose her name based on the Irish meaning of Brianna as "strong" along with her middle name Nicole, meaning "victory." Little did we know at the time just how appropriate the meanings of her names would be; how strong she would need to be in her life with her upcoming challenges to eventually achieve her victory. I have frequently reminded myself of what her name means, and I have also reminded her, from time to time, that her name is very meaningful and appropriate. There are no accidents.

My dad, a General Practitioner, was in the delivery room when Brianna entered the world. I hadn't been feeling too well, and was suffering from a cold and a sore throat when I delivered her. My dad had taught me self-hypnosis for the delivery, and everything went very smoothly during the quick four hours of labor. He was the first to see her and he chuckled and said, "You have a pistol there. In all of my years of delivering babies, I have never seen eyes like hers." I thought that he was just being a proud grandpa, however, he knew something was very different about this little baby who was wide-eyed and looking around with the attitude of "Where the heck am I, and who are you?" "A pistol" would become an understatement.

We only stayed 24 hours in the hospital before being released to go home. I don't remember much about seeing Bri during our hospital stay because I was quite sick with a cold, and the nurses had taken Bri away so that I could get some rest. When we got home, I was so excited to be a mom and I was looking forward to nurturing and nursing my new baby girl and bonding with her. I had always thought that nursing a baby was just a very natural thing to do. However, I would soon find out that not every mom and baby is natural at breastfeeding. Bri refused to nurse, and it soon became apparent that we needed help. I reached out to our pediatrician, and they set us up with a lactation specialist immediately. The specialist tried all sorts of things, but Bri had difficulty latching on. She was very upset and agitated with the whole procedure. The specialist gave me guidance and came back to check on us the next day. It was the weekend and we continued to work with the specialist, but it wasn't going very well. I was becoming frustrated and Bri wasn't too happy either. On Monday, we had our first visit with the pediatrician. We were horrified to find that Bri had lost a pound over the weekend, going from a very small baby of 5 lbs 6 oz to just 4 pounds 6 oz. The doctor and lactation specialist were determined that I was going to nurse my baby, but my husband and mother had other thoughts about it. When I got home, my hubby and my mom told me to feed my baby and if it took using a bottle to do it, so be it. Bri was starving and the lactation specialist was biased, so I didn't listen to her anymore. I started using a bottle and pumping breast milk to feed Bri. It took many tries with different nipples before Bri would actually latch on and feed. At this point, I was beginning to feel like an absolute failure, and I was brokenhearted; all I wanted to do was to bond with my baby, and instead, I felt like she was rejecting me.

Feeding seemed to be going alright with a bottle once we found the right nipple, however, we started noticing that Bri was quite agitated and difficult to calm. Our friends also had young babies and their experiences were quite different from ours. Their babies were nursing well, sleeping well and seemed to be happy. They were enjoying dinners out and visiting with family and friends. Bri wasn't sleeping well and had started crying all day and all night, so no dinners out for us, or visiting with family and friends. The pediatrician chalked Bri's discomfort up to being a colicky baby and instead of breastmilk, he suggested that we start her on a soy formula. She started to have projectile vomiting and then he suggested that we try Nutramigen, a nasty and foul-smelling concoction of brown goo. Needless to say, Bri didn't tolerate this formula either.

Back in 1991, there was a technique to get a baby to sleep through the night called the Ferber method. Dr. Ferber's technique had parents let a baby cry themselves to sleep for three nights in a row, and then they were supposed to sleep well from then on. You were to put your baby in their crib and if they cried, you were not to check on them, you were to let them cry it out and they would fall asleep. He said that it would only take three nights to get them used to falling asleep on their own. My husband and I gave it a try. It was heartbreaking and Bri screamed bloody murder the whole time. After two hours, she hadn't fallen asleep, and we went in to console her. We tried again the next night and the third night to no avail. So much for Ferberizing our sweet, but very uncomfortable baby, she was having none of it and it seemed cruel, so we didn't pursue it any further. Sleepless nights it would be.

Bri continued to cry day and night for nine months. We introduced solid food when advised to do so and it seemed to help a little. She started walking at around 10 months and immediately she turned into a completely different child. She seemed happier, although she still wasn't sleeping well, and she had also given up the little napping that she had done.

As Bri became a toddler, things seemed to improve, Her sister arrived 2 years later and all seemed well. We had play dates, swim lessons, dance lessons; we traveled, and had adventures with family and friends. I was starting to feel like motherhood might not be so bad after all. Bri's sister, Tara, was an easy baby who slept well, nursed well, and was a very content baby, like the baby that I had initially envisioned. Bri had become a gregarious toddler, and people gravitated toward her. It seemed that the worst was over.

Looking back, I wonder if Bri's first few months of being inconsolable were due to what we would later learn about her health. For the next several years, up until she was ten years old, I was under the impression that Bri was an active, athletic, healthy, happy child and that there was no stopping her. I had visions of her setting the world on fire, being a great student, and a leader. I observed her playing with her friends and thought how lucky she was to have a lot of great friendships. In school, early on, Bri had shown great potential and was placed a year ahead because she was doing so well academically. All seemed well.

Bri's Perspective

I don't have too many memories before the age of ten. What I do remember, felt pretty normal. I remembered fun family gatherings, playing with my friends, and having a fairly normal and fun childhood. The only weird thing I can remember is how all my friends could run around all day and never tire. When there was snow, they would run up the hill with sleds and slide down again and again. They could jump on the trampoline until they got sunburned from too much sun exposure. I thought everyone felt as tired as I did and were also just faking having the energy to play. Later in life, I realized most kids did indeed have that much energy.

2

A Mama's Perspective

My husband had worked for a very large construction company, and in 2001 we were facing a transfer from Kansas City, Missouri back to Texas. We decided that we wanted to go home to Colorado instead. We were missing family and we decided to move back to a small town, so that the girls could develop friendships before entering their teenage years. Other families that had previously faced transfers had advised us to try to keep things stable when our kids were entering their teenage years. Moving would mean leaving a large group of girlfriends in Kansas City, but we felt that moving to a small town would give us a lot of support and our girls would make new friends easily. Both my husband and I had lived in small towns, and we had really enjoyed the close-knit communities. We both had been welcomed into the small towns with open arms.

Our move to this particular small town would not be so idyllic. Instead, this town was very cliquish and didn't welcome new people with open arms. It would be very difficult for our two young daughters to make new friendships and even harder to join any athletic team in school because we hadn't raised our girls in this town. Only kids from town ended up on the sports teams. It became even more difficult when I went to enroll our girls in school and discovered that the 5th grade wasn't in the elementary school but was in the middle school. I was very concerned about this because Bri was a year ahead in school and very young to be entering middle school. My concerns would be well founded. This particular year, the middle school hired a special school psychologist to supplement the regular school psychologist because the girls in the school were just being horrible to each other. The drama was nonstop. Bri was constantly being brought into the psychologist's office to get her side of the story even though she was trying desperately to stay out of the fray. It got to the point that she was being taken out of class so frequently that I finally told the psychologist that Bri wasn't involved in the drama and to leave her out of it, no more taking her out of class to get her side of the story. Finding new friends was not going to be an easy task.

I started noticing that Bri wasn't as happy as she had been in Kansas City with all of her great girlfriends. I thought it was just going to take some time to make new friends and fit in. Bri had also started to complain that her muscles were "hyperflexing." Her dad and I thought that she was describing what we thought were growing pains. Her dad is 6'2" so we thought that she might turn out to be quite tall and that she was just growing. Along with her suspected growing pains, she was starting to have horrific nightmares. Our new home was large, and our two girls had chosen the downstairs bedrooms. There was a living room downstairs with a TV and Bri was so uncomfortable at night with the "growing pains," nightmares, and general insomnia, that she began to watch TV into the wee hours of the morning. Because she was awake and ready for school in the morning and seemed happy, I didn't think there was anything amiss until one night at 10 pm I received a phone call from a mother of one of Bri's friends. She told me that her son had just gotten off the phone with Bri and that Bri was suicidal! This came as a complete shock. We immediately went downstairs to find out what was going on. Bri told us that she was having difficulty with making new friends, she missed her old friends, that school was harsh, that her muscles hurt all the time, that she wasn't sleeping, and she was starting to have daily headaches. We stayed with her all night, and I was able to get an appointment with a counselor/psychologist for the next day.

Bri's Perspective

Boy did my happy childhood change drastically when my family moved back to Colorado. First off, I went from having a dozen girls our age on our street, to having one friend a few blocks away. This friend was always busy participating in sports and school studies, so I rarely saw her. I had another friend on the other side of town, but she was a popular athlete who would always cancel plans with me for other friends or boys. Middle school life was hard for me as most of my "friends" were not good people. I was constantly bullied and pulled into drama that I wasn't a part of. I tried all the sports I could during my four years at that middle school, but that was a dead-end as well. The fact that you had to grow up in the town to get any good coaching and the fact that I was easily exhausted made it difficult to play sports. My parents always wondered why I wouldn't go after the ball in team sports and why I couldn't keep up with the others in cross-country or track. They had no idea how physically exhausted I was during practice and games. I, once again, just thought that the other kids were tougher than me and I pushed harder, even though I honestly tried my hardest all the time.

Friends were nearly impossible to make as most of the kids would make up stories and talk behind someone's back. Even 20 years later, I don't get why people create drama. Even my nerdy group of friends would be full of drama. Why 12-year-olds cared so much about who-liked-who and who-did-what will forever elude me. One of my best friends stayed out of the drama. I think because she threw herself into her academics and sports. But this also meant that the best friend in my life was too busy for me.

My social life was a mess, but so was my private one. I started experiencing horrific nightmares and insomnia. My nightmares involved being abused although I had never consciously known of any abuse, and I wouldn't be able to fall asleep until 3 or 4 in the morning. I never told my parents because I knew they would blame the TV and suggest I just read. I was uncomfortable because my forearms, hands, calves, and feet started to ache and cramp. I kept the volume on the TV as low as humanly possible to escape being found out by my parents. I was uncomfortable, I couldn't sleep, and it was before cell phones or good internet so the TV was my only solace at the time.

I'm not sure why I thought the thoughts that I did in my preteens. I just knew I was miserable and tired. I knew that there was a way to end it all. As I went to do it, the phone rang. I let it ring through and told God if it was a sign from Him, to have it ring again. Sure enough, it did. It was one of my only real friends at the time and he said he had this big feeling to call me. I divulged to him that his feeling was with reason and what I was about to do. He told his mom who then called mine.

3

A Mama's Perspective

Bri started seeing her first counselor on a weekly basis. I was not present while they talked for an hour each week. Bri was still doing really well in school. Granted, she had very few friends but as a family we did a lot of fun activities like sailing, skiing, camping, hiking, rafting, flying with my parents, and traveling. We were close to both sides of our family. Bri's angst seemed out of character and out of proportion to the typical coming-of-age issues that kids face. I wasn't aware that Bri was being bullied at school.

Bri began having daily headaches and she would eventually be diagnosed with migraines too. She quietly dealt with her nightmares, not sharing with her dad or me that she was having them frequently and how horrific they were. She continued to have insomnia. By the time she was 13, she was starting to have episodes where she looked like she was shivering. They would last up to 20 minutes. My mom and I thought that maybe she was encountering a food allergy, so we started to try to work with her diet. Bri could "shiver" even when it was 90 degrees outside. I had also found out that Bri and some schoolmates would explore the old, abandoned sugar factory outside of town and I thought that maybe they had been exposed to toxic elements. However, when I asked the other parents if their kids were having any health issues, they all said no.

When Bri was 13, she had been seeing a counselor for over a year and nothing had changed. She was still miserable, having daily headaches and insomnia. Along with the shivering episodes, she started to have what I would describe as arm flutters. She would disguise the movements by playing with her long hair as her right arm involuntarily fluttered up and over to her right side where she'd grab her long hair quickly and twirl it. I wasn't aware that she wasn't just playing with her hair for quite some time. No one at school had figured out that she was having involuntary movements. Bri had joined the band and was a percussionist; she was vying for the second chair. Her coordination was amazing with her arms and legs playing independently. At this time, we decided to switch counselors and she was diagnosed with Post Traumatic Stress Disorder (PTSD) probably due to the nightmares. Cognitive Behavioral Therapy (CBT) wasn't doing much to alleviate her distress. The counselor tried Eye Movement Desensitization and Reprocessing Therapy (EMDR) and things seemed to improve for a while; or so I thought.

Bri's Perspective

My best friend at the time suggested I join the band with her as a percussionist. It was the only instrument you had to try out for because it seemed like everyone wanted to be a percussionist. Honestly, how could you disagree with that? Drummers are so cool. I tried out with her and made it. Drumming came naturally to me and I really enjoyed it. My best friend would practice drums every day along with her other endeavors. She was a skilled athlete, an A student, and had to be the best at everything overall. This didn't bug me as I never had to be the best. I was plenty happy being good at what I pursued without trying. She had been practicing with the band teacher in secrecy to play the drumset for months when of course she finally wanted to show off to me. I had never played a drum kit, but after she showed me what she had been working on for months, she told me to try. I got behind the kit and instantly picked it up. I played the same beat as she did within 5 minutes. I fell in love with drumming and I'm pretty sure she was a little agitated by this. All of our junior high years, she would practice day and night to be the best and I did a minimal effort just to come in second.

Around this time, I remember starting to have these weird jerks but I thought they were kind of funny. They didn't hurt. I couldn't control them and I could easily turn them into just playing with my hair or something. However, the muscles in my arms and legs began to constantly ache. I would wrap my arms and legs in ACE bandages and then wear long sleeves and pants to conceal it, because I didn't know how to explain what hurt or why it hurt.

The "shivering" was weird. We would later figure out that I was having tremors. I would be sitting and my whole upper body would just start to violently shake, as if I was super cold. My mom and grandma tried to throw jackets and blankets on me, but I swore I wasn't cold. I would just tremor violently for what seemed like forever. My grandma was positive I must be allergic to Monosodium Glutamate (MSG), a flavor enhancer, since she first saw me "shiver" at an Asian restaurant and she had bad reactions to it. She would often get heart palpitations. I also remember it happening at the theater, in cars, and random other places. The longest episode lasted about 20 minutes. These episodes didn't really hurt either, but they were pretty draining.

4

A Mama's Perspective

By 14, Bri was starting to have violent and lightning-quick jerking of her right arm. She could no longer hide the movements and kids at school were becoming aware of her jerks. They were bullying her even more. She had two girlfriends at this time, one was an athlete and the other was an academic all-star and athlete with a big heart. Both girls were extremely busy, so Bri didn't get much time to hang out with them and her isolation was increasing. She remained an A-student and an athlete, although her athleticism was in skiing, swimming and rock climbing, not school sports. She also became an avid motorcyclist. Our family skied a lot, I had no idea just how much she hated the cold and how exhausted she was during any physical activity. We didn't realize that cold temperatures set off her symptoms and her body hurt. She put on such a brave face and never complained.

With Bri's discomfort and cramping muscles, I thought that seeing a chiropractor/acupuncturist might help. She started seeing Dr. MS. Although the chiropractic treatments and acupuncture treatments weren't alleviating her symptoms, he was very caring and interested in helping her. She continued to see him for about two years. Also, around this time, I thought that maybe Eastern Medicine and Chinese Medicine might be helpful. After a few visits, we decided that it wasn't making a difference and she stopped seeing them.

Bri's Perspective

I didn't know what was going on with my body, just that I was getting more and more uncomfortable. We went to a chiropractor that was the best. He was sweet and handsome, and his hands melted into you. I so desperately wanted his treatments to work; I had a massive crush on him. I was also pretty open-minded so I was mentally trying to get acupuncture/chiropractic medicine to work. Alas, it did not.

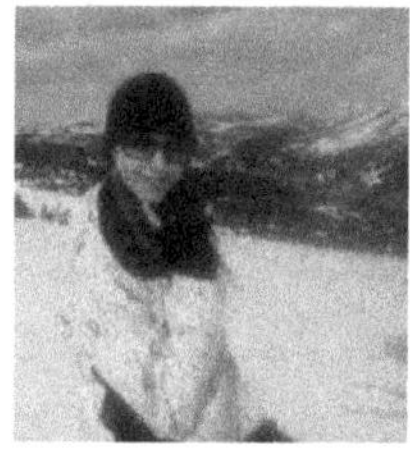

One of our many ski adventures

My family was born and raised in Colorado and loved snow sports. I tried my best to enjoy them, but the cold hurt my body, and the physical activity was exhausting. I thought that there had to be something to it as skiing and boarding are expensive activities, yet people keep doing it. Why would they spend that kind of money to torture themselves? I tried to force myself to like it. It never happened for me. As for school sports, I was terrible. My cross-country coach said I had the body of a runner, but I would always come in near last place. In track, I really wanted to do the long jump or sprints but because we were new in the small town, I would only get chosen for hurdles and relays. I also tried volleyball, basketball, and swimming, before I decided maybe sports just weren't for me. I ended up enjoying other activities like riding motorcycles, shooting, roller skating, skateboarding, drumming, and less physically intense activities.

5

A Mom's Perspective

As Bri's symptoms of weird movements became more apparent at 15, along with increasing anxiety and depression, I decided that it was time to see a neurologist for some answers. Her primary care physicians didn't have any answers. They had no idea what was going on with her irregular and involuntary movements that were becoming more frequent with more limbs affected. On both sides of our family the only neurological disorder was with my mom and my grandpa's Restless Leg Syndrome. Bri's grandma, my mom, had Obsessive-Compulsive Disorder (OCD) tendencies and was brilliant. My dad was also brilliant. Both were pilots, blue water sailors, entrepreneurs, and my dad was a general practitioner who had a photographic memory. Both of my parents were always on the go. My various family members having OCD and high intelligence would later lead to Bri being misdiagnosed. I also found a hypnotherapist. Knowing that my dad had great success with his patients using hypnosis for various things, I thought that by reaching Bri's subconscious we could turn things around and have her feeling much better. I had finally become aware of Bri's ongoing nightmare issues and insomnia. I thought that maybe hypnosis would be the answer to calm things down.

Bri's dad and I went with her to her first neurology appointment. Dr. MM asked a lot of questions and took a thorough history. He then ordered blood work to rule out Wilson's disease, Lyme and Rocky Mountain tick-borne illnesses, West Nile, and other conditions. I felt that the blood tests were extensive and that we might eventually get an answer. The blood tests came back normal. With the family history of Restless Leg Syndrome, Dr. MM thought Bri might also have RLS or possibly Idiopathic Hereditary Essential Tremor [idiopathic, meaning they don't know the cause.] He also mentioned the possibility of Myoclonus, a neurological disorder causing sudden jerking. Dr. MM had also ordered a Magnetic Resonance Imaging (MRI) which was normal. He prescribed Clonazepam, an anti-seizure medication, for Bri's involuntary movements to quiet them down. However, she was just 15, we really didn't have any answers. We weren't ready to put her on a benzodiazepine without knowing just exactly what we were dealing with so we declined the prescription. When we went to the front desk to schedule our next appointment, the scheduler informed us that Dr. MM was moving out of state and that his partner wasn't going to be taking on his patients. It was disconcerting to us because he had just prescribed a benzodiazepine with no intention of our daughter being followed by him or his partner. This would not be a good omen going forward. I looked up Myoclonus, and some of the symptoms were present like the lightning-quick jerking and twitches. However, I knew that Bri was also experiencing muscle spasms and cramping and Myoclonus didn't include these symptoms, so I wasn't convinced. The information on Hereditary Essential Tremor also didn't explain all of Bri's symptoms. [1,2]

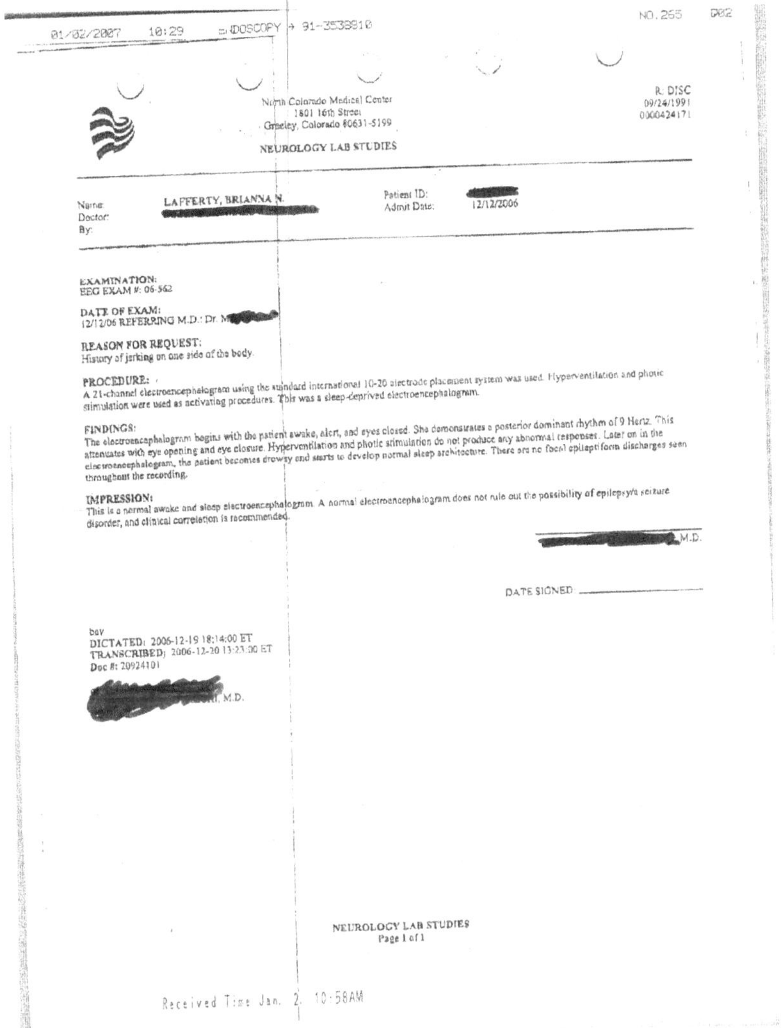

Neurology Lab Studies Report

Had Dr. MM not abruptly quit practice we might have had answers much sooner. From his notes and treatment plan, he was actually quite close to diagnosing Bri. This could have saved us so much anguish, time, misdiagnoses, and money. When his partner wasn't taking his patients, it really threw us for a loop. We had to start again with another neurologist. It seems that the universe was going to have a much longer journey for us. It wasn't going to be easy.

"Myoclonus refers to a quick, involuntary muscle jerk." Although Bri was definitely having myoclonic jerking, this also didn't adequately explain all of her symptoms, so I pressed forward with finding satisfactory answers in order to have her treated properly.

Bri's perspective

At this point, I was really starting to get uncomfortable and easily fatigued. I think the first specialist we saw gave me some good hope. He was onto something. I would later find out that the medicine he prescribed is a Hail Mary in my life, but it was upsetting that he would put me on something so potent just to leave his practice without providing ongoing care for me. This would set up an early distrust of the medical profession for both my mom and me. The normal results would start off being a huge sigh of relief. The only abnormal test I received was low iron which would stay constantly low despite expensive supplements. However, after more and more tests came back with normal results, the answer seemed further away than ever. We started to wonder if we would ever get an answer, ever get a solution. What is going on, how bad will this get, will it kill me? These types of questions were all starting to circulate through my young, teenage brain. The wait for test results started to become excruciating.

I wish I could say that I was always cheerful and hopeful, like I am nowadays, but being a teenager is hard enough as it is, and then throwing an undiagnosed and increasingly painful disorder on top of it got to me.

LAFFERTY BRIANNA-3-8-07 FU
Page 2

<u>IMPRESSION</u>:

1. Restless leg syndrome type disorder with the possibility of periodic limb movement disorder with some muscle aching and myoclonic jerks.
2. Low ferritin.
3. Headaches, which are likely tension-type headaches.

<u>PLAN</u>:

1. For her headaches, continue to work with Dr. Springfield.
2. For the restless leg syndrome/myoclonic jerks/myalgias, at this time she does not desire any other interventions. She should continue to work replacing her iron
3. Repeat a ferritin in 3 months and compare it to her previous one. The last time we checked it it was 19. Hopefully this Bioferritin will help increase her ferritin levels and we can monitor her symptoms.
4. She should call if the symptoms are bothersome. At this time it is not overly bothersome. We could consider a trial of a dopamine agonist, such as Mirapex or a benzodiazepine.
5. See her in follow-up in 3 months, sooner if needed. Again, prior to the appointment she will check a ferritin level.

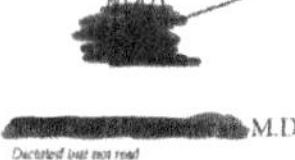

__________ M.D.
Dictated but not read

rm

cc:

MAR 1 5 2007

Centennial Neurology, PLLC
7251 W. 20th, Unit C ♦Greeley, CO 80634
Phone (970) 356-3876 ♦ Fax (970) 353-8810

Plan of Action notes

6

A Mama's Perspective

Bri continued to have ongoing symptoms that varied in frequency and intensity, as well as new symptoms. Along with her shivering (tremors), and right arm jerking, now her left arm and legs were starting to experience periodic jerking. Bri was still having "hyperflexing" muscles which we now know were muscle spasms and muscle cramps in her legs and her arms. She had been wrapping ACE bandages tightly around her arms and legs for several years and we had mentioned this to several of her neurologists but they didn't make anything of it. Many years later we would learn that wrapping her arms and legs tightly with ACE bandages was a sensory trick. By wrapping bandages tightly around an area, it alleviates sensation for a time bringing some relief. Bri had stumbled upon this sensory trick to make her muscles feel better for a short time.

For some reason, my mom mentioned that it looked like she was trying to fight something off. This really upset me. I think it hit a nerve because I knew by this time that my two daughters were experiencing paranormal activity in the house. Bri was complaining of nightmares and had started sharing that she was being attacked by evil entities. I know this sounds unbelievable, but we have since found reputable scientists, psychiatrists, and researchers that discuss these phenomena. As Mark Twain said[3] "The truth is stranger than fiction, but it is because Fiction is obliged to stick to possibilities; Truth isn't." It hit a nerve because I didn't have any tools to help my daughter defend herself against such attacks; yet I thought my mom might actually be on to something. It was very unnerving, to say the least. I wasn't able to confide in our church family. It was just too weird what was going on. By this time, I suspected that my girls were intuitives or possibly psychics, and our church viewed such things as toying with the devil. There would have been no support for us and the very real possibility of being shunned by our church family.

I looked at what both of our girls were experiencing as being their ability to access a wider range of frequencies; and the very real possibility of them encountering entities that reside in the wider range of frequencies. I liken it to a person who is color blind, they don't see much in the range of colors that most people do, possibly just black, white, and grays. Then there are people who see all sorts of colors, but not the range that someone with Tetrachromancy does because they have five cone types in their retina instead of three.

BANNER HEALTH COLORADO
Department of Medical Imaging
McKee Medical Center
2000 Boise Avenue
Loveland, CO 80538
MEDICAL IMAGING REPORT

Name: LAFFERTY, BRIANNA NICOLE   Physician: ██████ ██████ L.
MRN: 1069610   DOB: ██████   Pt. Type: O
Floor: OMR   Acct: ██████   EXAM#: 42A-052907
Room #:   Sex: F   Age: 15y Exam Date: 05/29/2007

Clinical Data: MYOCLONIC JERKS

Exam: SK MRI BRAIN W/O + W/CONT

HISTORY: Myoclonic jerks times 11 months.

TECHNIQUE: Sagittal T1, postcontrast FLAIR; axial T1 pre and postcontrast, FLAIR, diffusion; and coronal postcontrast T1 and FLAIR imaging was performed.

FINDINGS: Brain parenchyma is normal in appearance. There are no white matter lesions or mass effect or midline shift seen. The pituitary gland is mildly prominent with slight upward convexity of the tentorium. This is normal in a 15-year-old female. No focal pituitary lesions are identified. Infundibulum is midline. Prominent adenoid tissue is noted in the posterior nasopharynx, which is also normal for patient age. Orbits are unremarkable. Paranasal sinuses are well aerated.

IMPRESSION: Normal study. CLM/ms
DICTATED: 05/29/2007 19:36:21 ET
TRANSCRIBED: 05/29/2007 20:38:32 ET 290558/23987164/19039417

signed: ██████████ MD

Signed:
████████████

CC: ████████

Final Report

Page 1 of 1

First MRI Notes

Bri's Perspective

By putting pressure on or above the muscles that hurt and cramped, I would experience a type of distraction or sensation that alleviated the pain I was experiencing. While it never truly went away, it did help more than anything that I had tried. I think I found this "trick" by asking my sister to press on the muscles that hurt, or by pressing on them myself, which gave me some temporary relief. I figured the ACE bandages would be the closest to replicating the feeling of putting pressure on my sore muscles long-term. It was the only relief I could get for a while. My mom would later find a clinic on the east coast that was using tongue depressors in trials for cervical dystonias. We never made it to the specialized dentists that had videos on using the tongue depressors to see if the dystonic postures would cease, but we learned later that the tongue depressor trick was similar to my ACE bandage trick and would probably have done very little, if anything, for me in the long run.

Looking back on my medical notes which have been stored away for quite some time, my first doctor was on the right path. Had he stayed in practice we may have gotten some better solutions and answers way sooner than we did. He was on the right track by labeling my symptoms as RLS-like and myoclonic-like and with some of the medications he wanted to try. Without a firm diagnosis, these notes were ignored for many years to come.

Around this time, my involuntary muscle jerking had begun to get more violent and I would hit myself or objects around me. I would also start throwing whatever was in my hand at the moment. Once, I shattered a glass during myoclonic jerking. The shard I was still grasping went up and over my arm and body cutting it before I could let go. I also shattered a plastic cup grabbing water from the refrigerator. For obvious reasons, we started carrying insurance plans on my cell phones, because many times the jerks were so quick and violent that my cell phone flew out of my hand. On several occasions when I was in the car with my mom driving, I'd have a jerk and my cell phone would go flying, sometimes hitting my mom in the head. During bad episodes of myoclonus, I would not cook with oil or use any knives. After a couple of incidents that I ended up with burns, I stopped using a curling iron on my hair because it had become too dangerous to use during these episodes.

7

A Mama's Perspective

I scheduled an appointment with another neurologist, Dr. MJ. She had the notes from Dr. MM for the visit. She too thought that it might be Essential Tremors or Myoclonus based on Bri's history of symptoms. At this time, Bri's symptoms were sporadic and neither Dr. MM nor Dr. MJ had witnessed her movements during the appointments. Cellphones and their videography were still in their infancy stages so recording these movements and symptoms hadn't really crossed our minds. When Bri did experience symptoms she was pretty embarrassed by them and usually begged me not to record them. One of the things I wished I would have done early on would have been to have kept a journal of the doctor's visits and asked for copies of everything, like lab work and imaging, along with suspected diagnoses and treatment plans. I didn't realize what a journey this would become and I would only later start a journal, although still not a very thorough one.

Dr. MJ scheduled Bri for an Electromyography (EMG), a diagnostic procedure where they run electrical impulses through the muscles to test for nerve signal functioning. It can be quite painful. At our next appointment, Dr. MJ canceled the EMG and instead proceeded to tell us all about her troubles with her teenage kids. She actually brought us into her office and proceeded to pour her troubles out on us. She said to make another appointment which we did, but within two weeks we received a phone call from her secretary saying that Dr. MJ had left practice for "family reasons."

Again, not a good omen. I wasn't about to give up as Bri was becoming more and more miserable. I made an appointment with Dr. RP, another neurologist in our area. Bri was starting to fight me on seeing anyone else. She was still seeing a counselor who was using the EMDR technique that actually works really well for a lot of people, especially for those with PTSD, but it wasn't doing much to help Bri. Bri was also seeing a hypnotherapist without any relief. Of course, our insurance didn't cover any of these visits back then and we had to pay out-of-pocket for these services.

8

A Mama's Perspective

Bri had turned 16 and her symptoms were very apparent; she was feeling like an outcast. Going out to lunch, or dinner, usually ended up in embarrassment for her when a twitch, or a jerk, had her spilling her drink, throwing her food, or throwing her phone across the room. Everyone would stare at her. No one understood her, and she was becoming increasingly isolated. It didn't help that we had moved from the small town to a home on acreage about 20 minutes outside of town. She was excelling in her high school and she was enrolled in Advanced Placement (AP) courses. She was also running a burrito business, selling delicious breakfast burritos (Britos) to construction workers and classmates before school. However, she had very few friendships and would come home from school exhausted. Bri was still having insomnia, fitfully sleeping for only 3-4 hours a night. Her primary care physician had prescribed Trazodone for sleep when she was 15 but it never seemed to help. She was only taking 50 mg at the time. She also still had the occasional nightmares.

Dr. RP had Bri's medical history and he thought that her symptoms were indicative of Myoclonus. He had told Bri that she should stop skiing because she could fall off of the chairlift when she jerked. He told her with her seizure activity that she shouldn't swim anymore or ride her motorcycle. Bri was really upset with all that he was telling her she couldn't, or shouldn't, do anymore. I told Bri that we would risk it and continue our activities like normal and deal with the consequences if anything happened. I wasn't going to have a miserable and bedridden 16-year-old. Bri had too much she wanted to do, even though she was in constant pain and couldn't depend on, or trust, her body.

When I pressed him on the other symptoms, namely the muscle spasms and muscle cramping, he didn't think too much of them. She was also having a lot of nerve pain which she described as having "molten-fire hot ice picks" jabbed into her and that her body felt the nerve pain everywhere. She described it as what a Christmas tree all lit up with blinking lights would look like, the blinking lights being her various nerves on fire all over her body and going off in pain. Dr. RP prescribed Neurontin for her but within seven days she had gained ten pounds and was getting blurry vision, a serious side effect of the medication, so he had her discontinue it.

He scheduled Bri for an Electroencephalography (EEG), a test to measure electrical activity in the brain and to look for seizure activity. During the testing, she was without symptoms. I mentioned that anything cold would cause her to have myoclonic symptoms, so he ordered an ice cream which she ate while hooked up to the EEG. Almost immediately she started having a pretty significant episode of jerking and twitches but her EEG was normal. So, with her various physical and psychological symptoms becoming more prevalent but her MRIs, CTs and EEGs and lab work all being normal, Dr. RP was beginning to think her symptoms were psychosomatic.

During her third visit, he was going to perform the EMG, he asked her a few questions about her nerve pain and where it was located. As he was preparing for the test, he became frustrated and said, "Nerve pain doesn't do that, I am not going to do the EMG and I suggest that you see a psychiatrist." When Bri came out of the room and Dr. RP told me that we should see a psychiatrist, I could see the devastation in Bri's eyes. We left the office but Bri just stood outside in the hallway, shattered, staring off into space. She had heard that what she was experiencing was "all in her head" and that she was a basket case, a crazy person. She stood there for over 30 minutes as I gently tried to coax her to leave the hallway so that we could get into the car and go home where I could hold her and try to comfort and reassure her.

Her depression worsened after this appointment; I became very worried about her. I knew that seeing a psychiatrist wasn't a good idea, but at this point, I was at a complete loss. I hadn't really seen Bri cry except when she was an unhappy baby. She was now bottling up her emotions and wasn't crying now. Looking back, had either Dr. MJ, or Dr. RP, performed the EMG, it might have saved us from further diagnostic hell in the future.

A few days later, I had my dad do a quick neurological exam on Bri, one he would have performed for one of his patients in order to determine whether or not to send them on to a neurologist for further evaluation. He didn't find anything of importance, although neurology wasn't his forte. He had also been retired for almost 20 years and he didn't have any contact with any of his former colleagues to ask questions for us. Dad had also never seen symptoms like Bri's and didn't know what to think of them. I didn't tell him that I was going to have Bri see a psychiatrist because he would have been furious with me. He was a very conservative doctor. He really eschewed using psychoactive medications to treat his patients because he felt that the medications masked issues that needed to be addressed. He also knew the various dangers with taking psychoactive medications. I really should have listened to my gut and remembered how my dad felt about psychiatrists and their medications. It would almost cost me my precious daughter's life.

9

A Mama's Perspective

Bri was suffering from daily headaches and she was beginning to have frequent migraines. I scheduled an appointment with a neurologist who was a headache specialist and he prescribed Topamax as a preventative and said to try it for a year as it reduces the frequency of migraines. He also prescribed the injectable Sumavel, or Sumatriptan, which Bri hated. It made her shaky and she fell asleep for 24 hours afterward, but it made her migraines go away. It was super expensive, about $300 an injection and not covered by our insurance at the time. She still occasionally uses Sumatriptan, but in pill form. It is a lot cheaper and easier to carry if needed. She had tried Maxalt, Frova, Relpax to no avail. It seems that only Sumaritriptan/Imitrex does the job for her and sometimes it even requires a dose of Tylenol with Benadryl to get relief, a trick her PCP told her about when the Imitrex wasn't cutting the migraines completely. (Please do not add these medications unless you consult with your physician, do not take this "trick" as medical advice.)

Bri's Perspective

My early teens were somehow more of a nightmare than my preteens. I was an insomniac with constant pain, and horrific nightmares when I could sleep. Every time we got close to a possible answer - it would evaporate without a trace. I started having headaches in middle school and became accustomed to them. However, I started getting migraines more frequently and by high school they were incapacitating. I had started seeing, and leaving, different doctors by this point. I was losing a lot of hope. Along with the muscle cramps, the twitching, jerking, and the headaches, I had also developed nerve pain. This pain would pop up anywhere lasting from a second to days in all of my extremities. It felt like a bee sting, or just painful electricity running down my nerves. I got better at explaining it over time.

Imagine your body as a Christmas tree all lit up. Some strands with lights that are constant and some that twinkle. Now, imagine those lights are pain signals. This is how I describe my nerve pain, it is very visual so I hope people can grasp what it might feel like. It's also like having the mini shocks of pain here and there, or the long zaps of electric-like pain all along a nerve pathway.

At this point, I was over everything. The doctors, the diagnoses, the lack of solutions. I was getting more depressed. I was starting to be in pretty bad pain; I had little sleep. Now I was told to see a shrink. I had been seeing shrinks off and on since I was a kid; I knew that it was also a pointless endeavor. I was told that I shouldn't do any of the sports I tried so hard to enjoy. I shouldn't ride my motorcycle, I shouldn't swim, I shouldn't ski. Basically, I heard that I shouldn't try to live. They didn't know exactly what was wrong with me and yet I was already being told that I had to give up what little life I had at 16 years old. They didn't even know if it was a fatal condition or not, so I began spiraling into a deep depression. At the time, I didn't know that what I had wasn't fatal because it seemed to be progressing and getting worse and more frequent. My mom wasn't aware of my fear, my fear that I might be dying or become incapacitated. Maybe she too wondered if it was going to be fatal?

10

A Mama's Perspective

It took me a while to convince Bri to see the child psychiatrist but she eventually agreed to see him, under pressure. She just wasn't up for a fight; she was only going to go to please me and make me quit bugging her about it. She'd had enough of doctors and their inability to help her. I scheduled an appointment with Dr. RJ and sent over all of her records. I was present for the appointments. An important thing to mention here is that when we lived in the small town, our girls had both experienced some strange paranormal phenomenon. Both of my girls had been seeing spirits but hadn't told each other, although they had each shared with me what they were seeing. Tara, Bri's younger sister, didn't seem to see the scary, dark spirits that Bri did, although they both saw what they described as a very tall, slender, dark, evil man with a top hat and a cape who would really frighten them.[4] They also saw what they described as shadow people who lurked in the dark corners of the basement. When they were observed, they would disappear into the walls. Tara actually became so frightened that she ended up moving to a bedroom upstairs that was right next to ours. Bri remained downstairs all alone to deal with the malicious spirits, along with her continuing nightmares and insomnia. No wonder she was so miserable and even suicidal. We discovered that our two daughters have a wider range of frequencies available to them, so they have some interesting experiences. Earlier, I related the ability to access a wider range of frequencies with the example of seeing colors.[5]

During Dr. RJ's history intake, I told Bri that we might as well come completely clean and share that she had been seeing entities, the "shadow people." I honestly didn't know what to make of it but at this point I thought it was time to share. Along with seeing shadow people from the periphery, and her anxiety, depression, panic attacks, and increasing OCD history, he was beginning to get a picture of what was going on. Adding to this, Bri's insomnia and sometimes up to three days of no sleep whatsoever, while taking sleep medication, he looked at this as having "manic" episodes. With my family's overarching perfectionism, their OCD tendencies, their little need for sleep, Dr. RJ diagnosed Bri with Bipolar I Disorder, meaning with psychosis because she was "seeing" things. I was frightened for Bri and delved into reading everything I could on the disorder. Bipolar I Disorder was formerly defined as manic-depressive illness or manic depression. It is a mental illness and there are three types. Bipolar I Disorder is defined by manic episodes that last at least seven days, or by manic symptoms that are so severe that the individual needs hospitalization. Depressive episodes last upwards of two weeks. There can be mixed episodes as well. What I was finding was horrifying. I was really concerned for Bri and her future. With the lack of mental illness in our family, how could this be that Bri had a scary mental illness? I also didn't quite resonate with the manic episodes. Yes, Bri could have a lot of energy and not sleep, but it wasn't the mania that I had seen depicted in documentaries. Her depression seemed to be more situational instead of ongoing, so this didn't resonate either. However, I was at my wits end and just wanted relief for Bri, so I agreed to having her medicated, against my better judgment.

Bri had had various symptoms for six years by now. We had refused any medications, except for the headaches, sleep medications or a trial of Neurontin for her nerve pain. I had learned that people with Bipolar disorder must stay on their medications. Against my better judgment, and with my husband's frustration growing, we decided that we would allow her to be medicated. Dr. RJ started her on Seroquel, Risperdal, Topamax, and Synthroid and she was also taking Trazodone for sleep, plus her primary doctor had also prescribed Flexeril as needed for her muscle spasms. I think she was also prescribed Amitriptyline for depression or Wellbutrin. I was absolutely horrified by the amount of medication that she was prescribed at such a young age. It was April and she soon ended up in an almost catatonic state. She was really out of it.[6]

Catatonia is reported with psychotropic drugs, including Risperdal/risperidone, which Bri was taking at the time. Looking back, starting all of the medications at once was something that I should have never done knowing how my mom reacted to all sorts of medications. I should have demanded that Bri start just one medication until we knew if she was going to react to it, then add another one and wait to see if any interactions between the medications occurred, and then add another, and another overtime keeping a journal of information related to it all. However, she started all of them at once! I now see this as being very dangerous and I would highly recommend against starting the medications all at once.

Bri's Perspective

I grew up in a Christian home where I was taught God would heal you if you asked. I would pray and ask God all the time for relief, or at least an answer. As it became more and more apparent neither would come, I became angry with God. I asked what I had done to deserve this, what my parents had done to end up with a child like me, and why I was a constant disappointment. Answers never came even when I screamed at him. I wasn't the only one becoming angry with God, my mom was having her issues as well, even with deep prayer and expectations. She was taught that every verse in the Bible is a promise that we can claim and yet here we were, no answers, no relief, and things were getting worse. Our prayers seemed to be falling on deaf ears.

I was already tired of seeing doctors who didn't know what was going on, praying a test would show something, and then to have everything come back normal. The disappointment that came with all of it was more than discouraging, it was excruciatingly frustrating. I had given up fighting; and when my mom kept urging me to see a psychiatrist, I finally gave in. When he asked if I saw shadows I said, "Yes" (as I did in our small town home.) We explained that when I would have these rare bouts of energy, I was hyper and unstoppable, sometimes for days and without much sleep. These two factors got me the diagnosis of Bipolar I Disorder. In reality, I was hyper and energetic when I wasn't experiencing my pain and I felt good, much like a normal teenager would feel with their normal energy. Instead, more medications it would be, and at this point, I welcomed being numb.

"Once you're labeled as mentally ill, and that's in your medical notes, then anything you say can be discounted as an artifact of your mental illness."-Hilary Mantel

11

A Mama's Perspective

Bri had become bedridden from being all doped up on the strong prescription psychotropic medications. At one point, I called each of her AP teachers and asked if she would pass her semester. They all said that she had done enough work and that her work was excellent, so if she didn't turn in any other assignments she would still pass her junior year. I didn't believe them but she did in fact pass her junior year with a B average while being catatonic and bedridden. She wasn't able to go to school for the last two months and she was a zombie. I wasn't aware until years later that Bri had tried to overdose on her Flexeril. She took a bunch but woke up later, alive. I hadn't been aware of her overdose because she had basically been catatonic for several weeks. I had been checking in on her but she was sleeping almost 24 hours a day, so nothing seemed different. I wished I knew. It is heartbreaking to think that I wasn't aware of her despair; that we had almost lost her. I would have immediately taken action, gotten her the proper help, with the discontinuation of her medications and a second opinion. I would also later learn that she wanted to end her life because she felt that she had become too much of a burden on us and wanted us to get on with our lives. Heartbreaking.

Bri's Perspective

I had entered high school. I was determined to be invisible and I succeeded well at this goal. I made good, not great, grades. I tried to live as normal of a life as I could, in the background. Even when I needed a cane to aid in my mobility, I still remained fairly unnoticed.I helped paint a mural in the band hall and helped the photography teacher roll film in my spare time. I even sold burritos to the school store, until the business teacher wanted me to sell at a loss. I declined and ended that business relationship. My symptoms were progressing and doctors didn't know what was wrong with me, so they started to prescribe a ridiculous amount of medications. As I took more and more medication I became numb to both myself and the world.

Often I would hear my mom screaming that she couldn't take it anymore. She couldn't take me being in pain and not being able to do anything about it. I knew she was up all night, almost nightly, digging into research on the internet. I consumed her life and I knew it. I figured if I ended my life my family would be sad for a time but they would heal and stop worrying about me. I didn't know what else to do, either. I was miserable; they were miserable. I thought if I just went to sleep and never woke up, everyone would be better off. I took 12 times my normal dose of muscle relaxer, thinking I would drift off and die in my sleep. I woke up three days later, angry that I hadn't succeeded.

12

A Mama's Perspective

There was an occasion early on in her medicated state, before becoming catatonic, that she went to school with her medications in her backpack. During class, one of her classmates who was a well-known druggie got into her backpack and took some of her pills. He ended up completely passed out. Later, he asked her what she was on because it was some 'crazy stuff'. Bri told me about it, and I filed it away in my mental file, wondering just exactly what it was that she was taking. After two months of Bri not coming out of her room and being quite unresponsive, I had had enough and decided to find another psychiatrist.

I scheduled an appointment with a psychiatrist, Dr. SS. He was world-renowned for dealing with Bipolar disorder using a natural approach. He visited with Bri and said she was absolutely not Bipolar, and that he would wean her off of all of her medications. I felt like such a failure. I had allowed my baby to be medicated into oblivion. I hadn't known just how dangerous the situation had become until months later. After she had been weaned off of all of the medications except for the Trazodone for sleep, and some migraine medications, she told me what she had done with the Flexeril. I was shocked and horrified, how could I have missed her suicide attempt, her scream for help?

Bri's Perspective

I was on a crazy amount of medications that I knew would knock any normal person out. I may have bragged about this as some sort of badassery armor. Well, a classmate who was known for his genius, as well as his drug habits, got into my pill case. The fact that he helped me in that class and my general disregard for anything at the time meant I only cared enough to warn him about the dangers of taking the medications. I didn't have the energy to stop him, fight with him, or report him, but I didn't want him accidentally killing himself. I told him, "Be careful, I'm on some strong stuff." He talked to me a few days later saying, "What the hell are you on, I couldn't move for like 24 hours!"

I brushed it off as him being an idiot drug abuser. I would learn later that the various medications for Bipolar I Disorder had been ineffective because I didn't have this disorder. I would also learn much later that the various medications for my condition would also be ineffective at bringing relief for me. Medications being in-effective for this condition is not unusual in most sufferers. For some reason, others with this condition also have a super high tol-erance for all sorts of medications like muscle relaxers, painkillers, and other drugs. While there are a few reports of medications being effective for this condition, many report that they are not. I would also learn that taking medications for something you don't have, like Bipolar Disorder, can be very dangerous. This is why it is im-perative to have a correct diagnosis and if you don't feel that you are getting a correct diagnosis, do not be afraid to get a second, third, or more opinions until you get the correct answers and treatment.

13

A Mama's Perspective

By this time, I was starting to research into the wee hours of the morning, usually from 12 am to 3 or 4 am because I just couldn't sleep knowing my girl was suffering. I would be up several times a week. This was difficult for me because I am not a night owl. However, I was driven and I needed to find answers for my sweet girl. Back in the mid-2000s, there wasn't much available on the internet concerning Myoclonus, Essential Tremor, or other maladies that we were being told she had, or what I suspected she had but couldn't find any information on. I would dig as deep as I could, even perusing professional journals for their insight and research. I would get tapped out when I would encounter the need to be a medical professional in order to access the information or that it would require a payment or subscription. I recently Googled a PubMed article and just saw the excerpt of it. It required a payment of $39.95 to access the full article. Not knowing if the information would be relevant and helpful, I wouldn't pay the fee to find out. I would wait many years for some of the information that I was seeking on Bri's symptoms, and possible disorder, to be made available to the public.

At this time, I began using charts of Bri's symptoms and what seemed to make things better or worse, the frequency, location, type of symptom, and other data points to discern a diagnosis, or discount a diagnosis she had just received that didn't resonate. I was still working with the premise that Myoclonus was involved but I wasn't getting anywhere with the other symptoms of muscle cramping and spasticity. I also chalked up the psychiatric features of anxiety and depression as being a normal reaction for a young teenager in my daughter's position: suffering an unknown illness, pain, lack of diagnosis, and isolation. It hadn't occurred to me that the psychological features would also be a part of an overall disorder.

I would later learn about Occam's Razor, Afrin (March 15, 2016), the idea that the simplest explanation is more likely than one that is more complex. Instead of multiple disorders/syndromes, there is usually an explanation and a disorder that encompasses every symptom. So, instead of Bri having Myoclonus and mental illnesses of anxiety, depression, panic attacks, and then a muscle disorder of some kind, there might be a disorder that encompassed all of it.

It's my understanding that doctors are taught Occam's Razor in medical school, but so far, it seems as if none of the ones we encountered had put two and two together to find out what I was beginning to understand. I found it interesting, the lack of curiosity on Bri's specialists' part. It seemed as if they were too overworked, and narrowly focused, to go home and do some homework, or to ask colleagues about an interesting case. More than once, I felt that I was being viewed by Bri's doctors as interfering by Googling Bri's symptoms, in an attempt to understand what we were dealing with. I was trying to understand what we were possibly dealing with in order to have an educated conversation with her specialists. If the specialists weren't going to lift a finger to find proper answers, I sure as hell was. I would later learn and remind myself that doctors work for us, they are not on a pedestal above our understanding, they are just humans with specialized education but that doesn't make them infallible.

14

A Mama's Perspective

In my many hours, days, and weeks of research, I had stumbled upon a very rare and incurable neurological movement disorder called Myoclonus Dystonia, also known as Alcohol Responsive Myoclonus Dystonia in my ongoing search for answers. Bingo! The disorder not only had the physical features of the twitches, tremors (which we had called chills/shivers), lightning-quick and sometimes violent jerking or myoclonus, muscle spasms, muscle cramping, spasticity, torsion and twisting, but the disorder also had psychological features of anxiety, depression, OCD, panic attacks and alcohol abuse. Wow! I also learned at this point that there were specialists, neurologists with a special focus on movement disorders who are called Movement Disorder Specialists. I had very high hopes at this new prospect of having Bri see a Movement Disorder Specialist. I felt that effective treatment was just around the corner. Boy was I in for a nasty surprise.

Bri's Perspective

I had given up on a diagnosis or treatment at this point. Doctors and family believed it was all in my head, except for my warrior mom of course. What I was experiencing was weird and unusual.

My friends at the time tried to understand, but no one ever did. Sometimes I would hurt too much, or I would just be too tired to hang out which eventually lost me a lot of friends. I don't blame them, I too would tire of friends who were "too tired" to hang out and of someone who could make a spectacle of herself when out in public if her symptoms decided to put on a show.

I remember a fun evening with my friends when we were just hanging out at a friend's house. We were just playing games and being silly when I had an episode. It scared a couple of my friends while the others thought it was too odd for them. This was one of the last times I hung out with a group of friends for many years to come.

A Mama's Perspective

Around this time I found an in-person Dystonia support group that met at least once a month, about an hour from our home. The support group was fantastic, although Bri felt like an odd-ball. Everyone was 50 years old or older. Some were disabled and in wheelchairs while others were suffering from Cervical Dystonia with their heads craned over to their shoulders. Most were on disability and had full-time caregivers. It wasn't the picture of living your best life. I think it really depressed Bri to see what her future might look like but I really appreciated the group's insight and compassion. They were fascinated with Bri, her various symptoms, and how young she was.

There was a gentleman that had not attended for a while and when he came back, he showed us that he had had a very new surgery called Deep Brain Stimulation surgery (DBS.) He had a battery/neurostimulator placed in his chest like a pacemaker and two leads in his brain that put out electrical pulses. His head had been craned all the way over to his shoulder prior to his surgery. He was miserable, he couldn't drive, or see very well, and he walked a crooked path. After DBS surgery, his head was almost in the normal position and he had such a big smile on his face. He asked if we all wanted to see what happened when he turned off his DBS unit and we all said, "Yes." Seconds after turning off his unit, his head careened back over to his shoulder and we all yelled, "Turn it back on!" It was a fascinating situation to witness.

I filed this new technology away in my mental file for a later date. I did some research and found out that it was experimental for several disorders. Bri had not been diagnosed with Myoclonus Dystonia, but I noted that DBS was not identified as a possible treatment. It was being used primarily for Parkinsons and Cervical Dystonias.

15

A Mama's Perspective

During the 2000s, our insurance carriers, Anthem Blue Cross Blue Shield or Cigna, both supposedly excellent company health insurance plans, failed us miserably. In a five-year period, we were out of pocket about $100,000. We had to pay for everything ourselves, when our insurance failed to cover the doctor visits, the various tests like MRIs, CTs, EEGs, the frequent blood work, the weekly counseling visits, the weekly hypnotherapist visits, the chiropractic care, and the acupuncture treatments. Plus, the various supplements and expensive medications were not covered. There was a clause at the time that excluded "mental illnesses" being covered, ones like Bri had been diagnosed with, namely the anxiety, depression, panic attacks, OCD, and Bipolar. We tried to get the Bipolar diagnosis expunged from her records but no one was willing to do that. I doubt that alone would have helped, as she had been seeing psychotherapists for years. She had been diagnosed with anxiety and depression along with PTSD and panic attacks previously.

Through our Dystonia support group, I asked a lot of questions as to who people were seeing for care. A majority of them said Dr. RK, a movement disorder specialist. I made an appointment with him, confident that he would agree with what I had been finding, that Bri was suffering from Myoclonus Dystonia. I had all of Bri's medical records sent over and we waited the four months that it took to see him. My husband had only gone with us to the first neurologist appointments, and since decided his role was to be a good provider, provide access to great insurance, and support us through love and prayer. My husband decided to go with us to this visit. It took us two hours to drive to the doctor's office for the 1:00 pm appointment. Then we sat in the waiting room as the receptionist repeatedly told us that the doctor was seeing an emergency in the office. At 5:00 pm we finally were led back to the exam room. Dr. RK entered the room brusquely looked at Bri, ran a probe down her spine, when she twitched, exclaimed that she had PNES or Psychogenic Non-Epileptic Seizures from a Conversion Disorder. He directed us to make an appointment with his neuropsychologist for weekly appointments. He also stated that her twitches were in a "frequency/rhythm that was psychogenic," as if he had taken the time to measure how fast or slow she was twitching. He had not and EMG's had never been performed. Then without allowing us to ask any questions, he quickly left the room. We were in a daze. Bri had just been told, again, that everything was in her head. She had heard that she was crazy. It didn't help that her dad was at this visit where he was told that Bri was suffering from a mental illness. Bri felt that he just looked at her differently from that point forward.

We declined to make an appointment with the neuropsychologist because Bri was still in school. It would have required a four-hour round trip once a week, and an ungodly sum of money. Our insurance wouldn't have covered the visits. Bri had been seeing a counselor weekly for years, along with a hypnotherapist, with no relief. We wondered what in the world would a neuropsychologist be able to do except keep us coming weekly, while charging a lot of money to do so. Bri would have been prescribed a bunch of psychotropic medications and some of their side effects were known to cause Tardive Dyskinesia, another movement disorder. We didn't need the psychoactive medications complicating things. The last attempt at medicating Bri for Bipolar was a complete disaster. I was also not convinced of his diagnosis of PNES. I was concerned that he may have seen the various misdiagnoses of Bipolar I Disorder in Bri's medical history. Combined with the PTSD diagnosis, anxiety, depression, and panic attacks and caused him to have a biased opinion.

16

A Mama's Perspective

I have since learned that many specialists have very significant biases and will diagnose what they seem to specialize in, or are more familiar with; a sort of tunnel vision. At the time, Bipolar was a very common diagnosis. This particular doctor was focused on psychogenic disorders: he had written articles regarding this type of disorder. I learned that Bri was extremely anxious for this visit. As we sat in the waiting room, it added to her anxiety. Her myoclonic jerks were set off by stress and she was feeling stressed. Dr. RK ran the probe down her back, but this was in tandem with her symptoms going off from her increasing anxiety. Her jerks were bound to show up with the amount of anxiety she was feeling. She continued to jerk all the way home from the visit. [7,8]

Considering Bri had been dealing with symptoms for several years, it didn't make any sense that her symptoms hadn't resolved and were, in fact, progressing. As you can see from what we have described, Bri didn't experience any numbness, paralysis, deafness, blindness, stuttering or extreme behaviors. However, Conversion Disorders are known to occur after significant stress, or emotional, or physical trauma. Bri was suffering from stress, however, Myoclonus Dystonia could be the source of her stress causing the psychological features of anxiety, depression, panic attacks and

OCD symptoms. There was a disorder that could explain all of her symptoms. Plus, the age of onset for her symptoms were consistent with Myoclonus Dystonia and she hadn't experienced any traumas, or stressful events, prior to her symptoms appearing at 10 years old. Her symptoms came on slowly, not abruptly like PNES. Conversion Disorders usually have a median onset age of 37-50 years old whereas Myoclonus Dystonia begins in the first or second decades of life just like what we witnessed with Bri.

From my perspective, the Functional diagnosis from a Conversion Disorder didn't make any sense to me for Bri and her history. I had found Myoclonus Dystonia which seemed to explain everything that we had experienced. I also looked into Psychogenic Non-Epileptic Seizures and made a comparison chart of what these symptoms would look like versus what Myoclonus Dystonia symptoms would look like. I checked off way more symptom boxes with the Myoclonus Dystonia and could discount various symptoms of the PNES from a conversion disorder. Also, with Bri having had years of psychotherapy, to no avail, and having been on psychoactive medications without relief, I just wasn't convinced by the PNES diagnosis, although Bri having psychological diagnoses weighed on my mind.

Bri's Perspective

Going to the dystonia group was insightful, but none of them looked how I looked or acted how I acted. My muscle spasms were in my arms and my legs and I twitched. Most group members had it in their neck with no twitching. Most of the group were older people, too. I was in my teenage years. I think we were told there was another young person but we only went a few times as it was pretty far away and I wasn't sure what help it provided. Through this though, we got the name of another doctor.

I was so hopeful for this appointment with Dr. RK as he was a renowned movement disorder specialist. I was thinking he could finally figure out what was wrong with me. We had waited months to see him and my dad had finally taken off time from his busy career to join one of these seemingly never-ending appointments. I remember feeling so guilty that he was taking time off of work to sit and wait for this doctor as all of my previous appointments had gone sour. I was getting really anxious. Finally, after four months of waiting to see him, an hour's drive, and 4 to 5 hours of sitting in the waiting room after our scheduled appointment, we got to see this "expert." He spent 10 minutes with us, ran a tool down my spine and I jerked. Because of this sudden reaction, he diagnosed me with PNES and suggested we talk with a neuropsychologist. He refused to listen to, or answer, any of my parent's questions. Once again I was devastated. This would temporarily destroy my father's and I's relationship. For a while, it seemed to change the way he interacted with me. He seemed to get more distant and would force me to get up and do things even though I was exhausted. I thought it was because he had heard that everything was all in my head and that I needed psychiatric help, I had a mental illness, and I was just trying to get attention. I would soon decide to make a plan to get out of the house and live on my own so that I wouldn't have to deal with my dad when I wasn't feeling well. By living on my own, if I wanted to try to sleep at weird hours, I could. Or, if I didn't have the energy to do something, it was my life and I could do what I wanted when I wanted.

I have since written to Dr. RK about how detrimental the visit with him was. As expected, he has not responded. He was arrogant then and I assume he still is. However, writing and sending the letter was cathartic for me. I have also gotten my dad's view of this particular appointment. I didn't realize my dad saw straight through him and didn't say anything on the way home because he was quite disgusted by the arrogance of this doctor. I thought the silence was because I was still twitching after being told it was in my head. I was trying so hard to hide the continuing twitches and I was so mad that I couldn't stop. I remember trying to keep the tears from falling and my cries from making noise. Looking back, we were out of answers. We had all tried to do what we thought was the best. His demeanor seemed like he believed what Dr. RK said when after talking to him; I think he was just confused and hurting, like we all were. He was devastated that we had not gotten answers.

"Opinion has caused more trouble on this little earth than plagues and earthquakes."-Voltaire

A Mama's Perspective

We went home in silence. I have since asked my husband what he was feeling during and after the appointment. He says that he was extremely disappointed in the visit. We had waited a long time for the appointment with a specialist that had come highly recommended, although he really didn't see anyone who was younger like Bri. Dr. RK mostly saw elderly patients with Parkinsons and Essential Tremor. We waited in the waiting room for several hours just to be given a few minutes of Dr. RK's time. My husband actually thought that the doctor thought we would tire of waiting and leave and he wouldn't have to see us. After a brief 10 minutes, we were given the diagnosis that was unsatisfactory, in our judgment. My husband was also very disappointed that we were not able to have our many questions answered.

We had been seeing specialists for years now and really wanted to understand what was going on. My husband became frustrated and really didn't know what to say. Articles claim that a knowledgeable neurologist will be able to differentiate between PNES (which can mimic an organic movement disorder like Parkinsons, Myoclonus, Dystonia, and Essential Tremor) and an organic movement disorder. Dr. RK didn't do any evaluation except run a probe down Bri's spine, he did not do his job. He wasn't interested in testing her for an organic movement disorder and came in with a preconceived, albeit, wrong diagnosis.

With PNES, there seemed to be a sudden, and later, onset for symptoms, usually in adulthood but not always, and some sort of emotional or physical trauma causing undue stress. I found that people's eyes blink rapidly, which Bri never did, and they tend to bite their lips, which Bri never did. Their movements with their arms or legs are less consistent with their pattern being incongruent, not fitting a recognized pattern. There also seems to be fainting, blindness, paralysis, deafness and more bizarre behaviors with the PNES. Sometimes an individual will respond to a placebo, and yet Bri had not had relief with real medications or alternative therapies. I would try to distract Bri to see if her symptoms would disappear and they didn't. In fact, I would hide and Bri wouldn't know that I was observing her and yet she would be in a full-blown episode of jerking and twitching, unlike what PNES individuals do, they usually display the behaviors in front of others. I also had witnessed Bri cutting her arm and body when the glass she was holding broke by hitting the corner of the countertop during a violent jerk. The remaining shard had cut her. PNES sufferers avoid harming themselves. The PNES diagnosis also didn't explain Bri's muscle cramping, spasticity, or nerve pain but Dystonia accounted for these symptoms.

17

A Mama's Perspective

At this point, Bri stated that she wasn't going to see another doctor…ever! I, however, had a much different plan. I wasn't about to give up, especially knowing that I was now onto a diagnosis that might be what Bri was suffering from. Unbeknownst to her dad and I, Bri had been drinking socially with her friends and her friends' parents. She realized that alcohol made her Myoclonic symptoms go away for a period of time. She could fit in and seem normal. She started drinking at around the age of 15 at her friend's house and probably ours as well. I think this also might explain why we would see an alleviation of her symptoms at times, while other times they would be significant. She had most likely been drinking when her symptoms seemed to "improve." The alcohol worked to alleviate the symptoms for a while.

Bri's Perspective

I had started to consume small amounts of alcohol with friends and noticed it basically cured my nerve pain, my twitches, and muscle cramps. I could focus better, and overall, be more human. The doctors and the drugs didn't work so I started drinking a little here and there. The alcohol seemed to work better than any drug we had tried previously. Towards the end of high school I was able to drink more and sneak it to sleep or to get through the day. I was always friends with the older kids or the kids whose family wouldn't mind buying it for us. Close friends knew it helped so I tried not to make it noticeable, but I had started to consume more than your average high school partier, even though I never went to any parties. Around this time is when I thought, 'I might as well do what I can' because the doctors can't help so I'll try my best and do what I need to do in order to survive.

18

A Mama's Perspective

"Keep trying; failures increase the probability of success."-Ken Poirot

It took me quite a while to decide on who to see next. The previous doctors had all been a bust and it was starting to look like I was doctor shopping which will get you stigmatized, making it very difficult to receive proper care. We were definitely verging on being labeled. I still thought that a movement disorder specialist was the one to see. I researched as best I could and I came up with a neurologist/movement disorder specialist who was also a professor at the University of Colorado at the Anschutz campus in Aurora. I made an appointment. I had to beg Bri to go. I decided that I wasn't going to be sending any medical records ahead of time as this seemed to pigeonhole Bri into a mental illness diagnosis. I was convinced that her disorder was not a mental illness but a neurological movement disorder. We needed someone to see her with "fresh eyes." I don't think that I would be able to pull this stunt off today with all of the electronic medical records where it seems everyone has access to your medical history information. I thank God for this blessing, that Bri was able to have a "fresh" appointment without prejudice from previous misinformation in her medical records.

When the day arrived for our appointment, Bri was definitely having a lot of very apparent symptoms. I still hadn't taken any videos of her movements. Dr. ML spent over an hour with us and she videoed Bri walking down the hallway. Then she witnessed Bri jerking her elbow into the corner of the countertop that she was seated next to. This alone convinced Dr. ML that this wasn't a psychogenic disorder because people with a psychogenic disorder usually will not harm themselves during their movements and Bri was definitely bashing her elbow into the corner of the countertop in a violent, myoclonic fashion.

After a few jerks colliding with the countertop, Dr. ML couldn't take it anymore and moved Bri to a safer location in the room where she couldn't hurt herself. She took a very detailed history and then asked if Bri had tried drinking alcohol and if so, what the effects were. Bri admitted that drinking alcohol alleviated her myoclonic symptoms for a time. Dr. ML then told us that the alcohol response was a diagnostic feature for Myoclonus Dystonia, otherwise known as Alcohol Responsive Myoclonus Dystonia. I felt relieved, finally a specialist who knew what was going on. She also diagnosed Bri with Myoclonus Dystonia due to the history of the physical, as well as psychological symptoms.

However, it wasn't going to be that easy. Dr. ML said that she had never seen a case of it in person and that it is extremely rare, even for the dystonias. She printed out a one-sheet piece of paper with the description of Myoclonus Dystonia on it and she said that I might try to research it but there wouldn't be much information available. This was in 2010. She also said that her colleagues had never seen a case of it either.

Dr. ML also wanted to have a genetic test run; the SCGE or sarcoglycan epsilon gene for a mutation that causes the disorder. It's also known as DYT11. The information that I have found suggests that 30-50% of Myoclonus Dystonia is caused by the DYT11 mutation and then there are a few groups of genes known to cause MD but it's a very small percentage. A more recent gene is the DYT15 but at the time it wasn't known. There's the KCTD17 gene that has an atypical presentation of Myoclonus Dystonia. Around 30-50% of the cases are due to mutations in the SCGE gene that provides instructions for making a protein called epsilon sarcoglycan whose function is unknown. This protein is commonly abundant in the nerve, brain, and muscle cells but a mutation in the SCGE gene causes a deficiency in the protein. This protein seems to affect the regions of the brain, like the cerebellum and basal ganglia, which are involved in the coordination of movements. In cases where the SCGE gene is mutated, it is inherited in an autosomal dominant pattern meaning one copy of the altered gene in each cell is enough to cause the disorder. It is usually inherited from the father but not always.

The rest of Myoclonus Dystonia cases are considered "idiopathic" or have no known origin at this time. Again, our insurance failed us and we ended up paying over a thousand dollars for the genetic test but we felt that it was worth it. No one on either side of our families had any movement disorders except for my side with the restless legs. We waited several months and when the results came back they said, "Inconclusive, de novo, spontaneous mutation." Dr. ML explained to us that it was going to be nearly impossible to locate where the mutation was. There was a possibility that it was a spontaneous mutation, and that is why none of our family members showed any signs of a movement disorder. I had found through my research that there seems to be more of Myoclonus Dystonia in Irish families. Both my husband and I have a lot of Irish ancestors.

We had this test done in 2010; her doctor said that it wasn't necessary to pursue any further genetic testing as it wasn't necessary to have the mutation to be diagnosed with Myoclonus Dystonia.

Dr. ML then proceeded to prescribe the various cocktails of medications used to treat Myoclonus Dystonia. She prescribed an anti-seizure medication called Depakote, but within a month Bri had gained 30 pounds on her very slight frame of only 100 pounds. I asked for it to be discontinued. Then she tried Keppra and within two weeks she was suicidal. So again, Bri discontinued the medication. She was put on an antidepressant of Buspar, a muscle relaxant of Flexeril, she was still taking Trazodone for sleep, and benzodiazepines like Clonazepam, Ativan, or others. Baclofen was not offered and neither was any dopa medications like Sinemet or Carbidopa/Levodopa.

19

A Mama's Perspective

During Bri's last appointment with Dr. ML we discussed how the medications were not working and what our options were. DBS at the time was experimental for Myoclonus Dystonia and Dr. ML wasn't willing to approve the surgery. She reminded us that Bri had Alcohol Responsive Dystonia and then she suggested that Bri could, "Drink if it helps and keep the drinks to 14 per week." [9]

I guess I started to look at alcohol as just a different type of medication. I had been told that it worked really well for this disorder because it is a Central Nervous System depressant, but when I told my husband what the doctor had told our 18-year-old daughter, he was furious. In Colorado, it wasn't legal for our daughter to purchase alcohol. I didn't know what to do. It was going on eight years of symptoms, many misdiagnoses, and many medication nightmares with no relief in sight. I was also very naive about alcohol because no one in our extended families had any substance abuse issues. I had seen the page describing Myoclonus Dystonia and its symptoms, including alcohol abuse, but I just never thought it would happen to us. I thought people had to have a propensity for drinking, like a family history of drinking in excess. Naive me, with Myoclonus Dystonia there IS the propensity to drink! Bri was living on her own by this time and she could access alcohol with her older boyfriend. She was going to school and working full time.

Myoclonus Dystonia is unique from the other movement disorders with the characteristic that alcohol can often result in a dramatic decrease in both the myoclonus and dystonia symptoms. It is also now being investigated that the alcohol abuse that stems from Myoclonus Dystonia and self-medicating might not be the entire story. When Bri was first diagnosed in 2010, her specialists weren't aware of the inherent danger in advising, "Drink if it helps." They also said, "Be careful," but we now know that because of the psychological features of this disorder it isn't that easy to just be careful. Once their brain has the alcohol it is extremely difficult for them to manage how many drinks they ingest and they don't seem to be able to control the amount of alcohol they consume, so they spiral into abuse whereas a lot of people can manage their intake of alcohol all throughout their lives.

There is something different about the Myoclonus Dystonia brain and its reaction to alcohol. Because the disorder has the Obsessive-Compulsive component to it, alcohol abuse issues may also be due to the compulsive aspect of the disorder and the difficulty for individuals to drink in moderation. We saw this with Bri later on when she had blood alcohol levels of 0.4 and was binge drinking. These are absolutely deadly levels. I should have been suspicious when we got a call from her boyfriend that they had been at his parent's house for a family dinner when Bri had too much to drink and was taken by ambulance to the ER. I thought it was just a case of being in the mountains at a high altitude with her low body weight of just 100 pounds and that she had overdone it with the wine. [10]

Bri's Perspective

Finally, I had a doctor who knew what was wrong! Sure, she didn't know what to do about it, but she admitted to that and did her best. When she asked if I had tried alcohol, she explained that she suspected Alcohol-Responsive Myoclonus Dystonia, meaning alcohol would settle down my symptoms. She told us about twins with the condition and how when they gave one twin alcohol, his symptoms would disappear for a while. While alcohol seemed to help, she was weary of this advice and told me I could drink if it helped, but to be careful. That advice is telling a person in severe pain who has insomnia, OCD, and anxiety that they have unlimited access to painkillers and sedatives (basically the alcohol and its effects.) On top of that, that person is a teenager with an immature brain, that just got the advice to drink if it helps and it sure did.

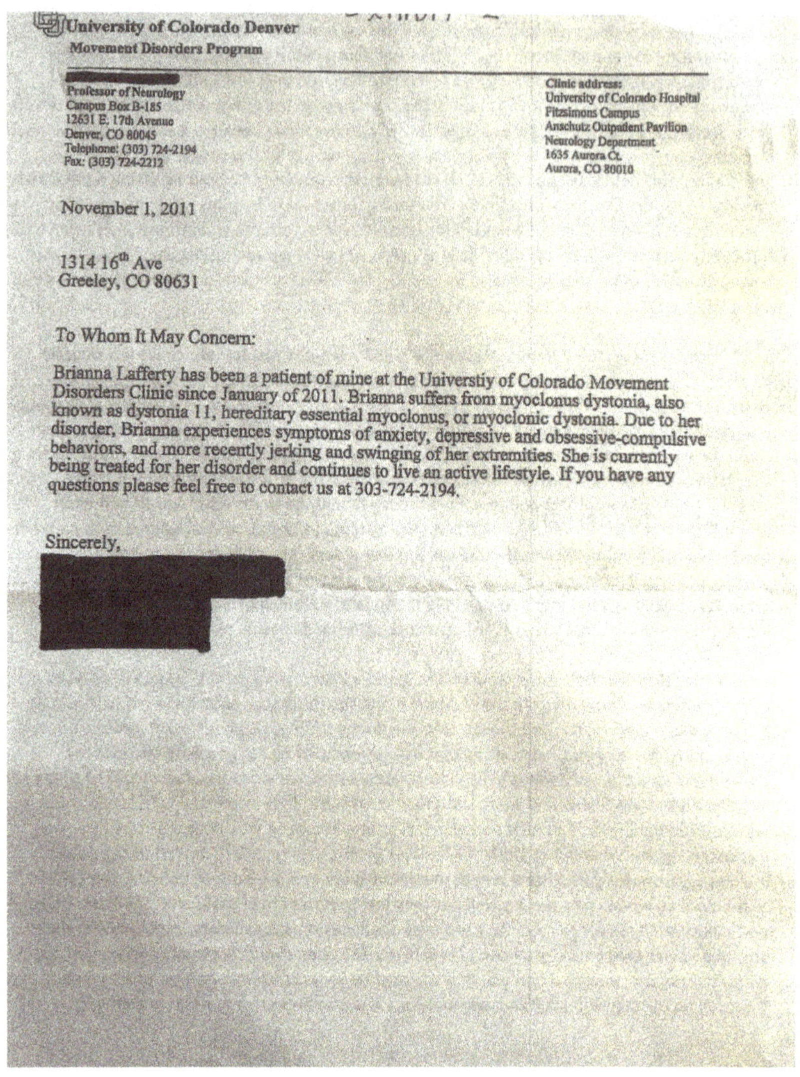

University of Colorado Denver
Movement Disorders Program

Professor of Neurology
Campus Box B-185
12631 E. 17th Avenue
Denver, CO 80045
Telephone: (303) 724-2194
Fax: (303) 724-2212

Clinic address:
University of Colorado Hospital
Fitzsimons Campus
Anschutz Outpatient Pavilion
Neurology Department
1635 Aurora Ct.
Aurora, CO 80010

November 1, 2011

1314 16th Ave
Greeley, CO 80631

To Whom It May Concern:

Brianna Lafferty has been a patient of mine at the Universtiy of Colorado Movement Disorders Clinic since January of 2011. Brianna suffers from myoclonus dystonia, also known as dystonia 11, hereditary essential myoclonus, or myoclonic dystonia. Due to her disorder, Brianna experiences symptoms of anxiety, depressive and obsessive-compulsive behaviors, and more recently jerking and swinging of her extremities. She is currently being treated for her disorder and continues to live an active lifestyle. If you have any questions please feel free to contact us at 303-724-2194.

Sincerely,

Diagnostic Letter

The above letter is the diagnosing letter that Dr. ML provided for me so that I could use it if needed with my professors, employers, or other specialists. It has been quite helpful on several occasions.

I was living on my own and not sleeping but I would fill my time with working and working out. My boyfriend and his family were all alcoholics so I would drink with them, but it wasn't more than once a week. I got into trouble when I went on vacation with them and thought I could drink like they did. I loved rock climbing and my boyfriend was an avid rock climber. Most of our time spent together was rock climbing. He wouldn't accept me having any medical problems so I pretended I didn't suffer from them. Climbing was exhausting but the mental and physical challenge was addicting. For some reason, I didn't cramp or twitch while climbing either so I could get lost in the activity for hours.

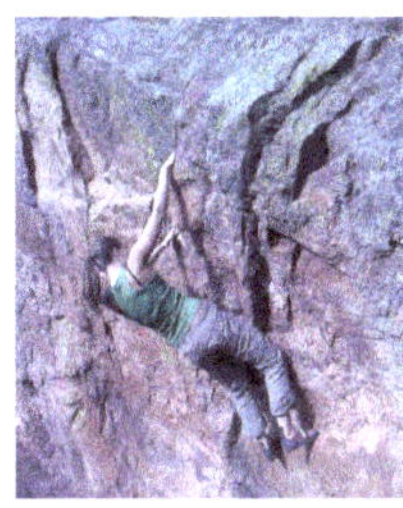

Rock Climbing
(Bouldering)

Looking back, it was probably a similar sensory trick much like the ACE bandages and drumming were - in other words, giving my overfiring signals a good place to go. The stretching and pressure on my muscles possibly worked as a sensory trick. I loved climbing, it was me and the next move in front of me. You couldn't worry about how long it would take, what 10 moves from now would look like, what you left behind you - only on the very next move. It was freedom and I felt alive.

I still wasn't drinking too heavily at this point, just the occasional few beers with my boyfriend. I couldn't obtain it otherwise being underage. It wouldn't be until I started staying at his house and camping with him that I began to binge a little. Everyone in the house did it, so I thought it was perfectly normal for someone my age. Instead of going to parties, we would just drink a lot at home, or camping, and all of us seemed functional. We never missed a day of work or acted in a way I thought was cause for concern. My parents thought I was functioning pretty well and thought that things might settle down.

20

A Mama's Perspective

At 19, Bri purchased a fixer-upper house and broke up with her boyfriend when he didn't show any interest in her purchase or celebrating with her. He had his own demons with drinking too much, so I wasn't too upset that they had broken up. She was still attending college although college was a lot different than High School. In High School, her teachers were accommodating and understanding, but in college, even with a letter of her diagnosis, her professors would not give her any accommodations. She was getting good grades in business courses. She also worked long shifts as a server at Red Lobster. Around this time, I had taken her to a Functional Medicine doctor; he suggested that she try a gluten-free diet. I thought that the change in diet had caused her symptoms to go into remission. I was not aware of how much alcohol she was consuming; that it was the alcohol that was keeping her symptoms at bay.

Bri's Perspective

When I was 19, I wrote a small description of how I was feeling; we found it looking back at our resources for this book.

"This is a letter I wrote to myself (or anyone who might be curious) as to what I was feeling and experiencing: "Would you like to know what's going on inside my head? I'm trying the hardest I can to hide what I feel from the world's eyes. Not just the shaking, the tremors, the tripping, the twitching; but the pain, the embarrassment, the worry, and the doubt. I'll explain. Here's a list of my symptoms. First, I will list all of them whether they happen all the time or not. Twitching, shooting pain, muscle aches, muscle fatigue, body fatigue, mental exhaustion, insomnia, muscle cramps, tremors, tingling in my fingers and my face, numbness in my fingers, daily headaches, migraines, insomnia, dizziness, nausea, vomiting, tripping, I can't put sentences together, acid reflux, pain behind my eyes. This is a list I quickly came up with that may even be missing one or two physical symptoms. I have been doing pretty well about not letting it wear on mentally, but as the symptoms get worse and as it begins to interfere more with my day to day life, it has become more and more draining mentally as well. Out in public on dates, I get embarrassed because I'm a young, healthy looking girl with twitching. It looks ridiculous and nobody is used to seeing a healthy person move in such a manner. I'm nervous for work when meeting people because I wonder, what if I twitch in front of them? How do I explain myself? Do I explain myself? How does

that affect a business relationship? At home, I have spilt water and broken glasses. What do I do if I am a guest at someone's home? What do I say? How embarrassing. Do I ask for accommodations ahead of time like needing a plastic cup or not helping with cooking if it requires using knives or hot oil? The myoclonus jerking has become dangerous to me and others in a few different ways. First off, the muscle contractions are so violent and forceful that when I hit something like a corner of a wall or a piece of furniture, it leaves huge bruises. I've also been hitting myself during episodes and leaving bruises. I can also break whatever it is that I hit. The muscles contract in unnatural positions which are very painful. If I try to control the jerk by tensing certain muscles, it puts pressure on different muscles causing unnatural positions too. It pulls in ways that are painful and it ends up hurting my joints and muscles. The myoclonus is also dangerous in the kitchen. If I have boiling water, or hot oil on the stove and I jerk, I could potentially spill the hot liquids on me or others around me causing severe burns. Knives are also potentially dangerous because one of my jerking movements has the motion of my right hand moving up and over my neck area or down my other arm and I am at risk for cutting myself or violently flinging the knife where it may cut someone close by. Driving is another potential danger if I were to jerk violently and pull the steering wheel without letting go briefly and quickly. So far, I have been able to sense it just nanoseconds before a violent jerk and plan for it. As a passenger in a car I have flung my phone and hit my mom in the head several times which could have caused an accident. As for the mental aspects of what I am going through, every symptom seems to be getting worse and I'm scared. I don't know what it means and I don't know what is going on. I'm trying my hardest to keep a normal life; taking care of myself, holding a full-time job, even taking care of my sweet dog Bean who also has seizures. I'm terrified things are getting worse and it's really hard right now to function "normally". I feel like Sh%& every day. Some days are better and some days are worse and I don't know how I'm not downing a bottle of pain killers just to get through the day (although pain killers don't do much for me so I don't take them.) I need sleeping pills to get through the night and yet they don't work all that well. When I get up in the morning, I have to plan my day out by "spoons". I'll explain. Let's say you have 15 spoons of energy per day. Each spoon represents the amount of energy it takes to complete a task. Brushing your teeth=1 spoon of energy. Taking a shower=1 spoon. Getting dressed=1 spoon. I only have 15 spoons for the entire day and I have to get up early to get ready for work, go to work, and make sure that I can make it home and eat dinner and get ready for bed. Some days I have more spoons than other days. It seems like I am getting less and less spoons per day because the symptoms are getting more frequent and worse. So, to be honest, I am terrified as a 19 year girl about what I can and can't do during the day. I don't know if I'll have enough energy to cook dinner, or how to hide this from people when it's getting to be more and more obvious. How am I going to keep going when I hurt more and more? I have a ton of questions, and so far, no great answers. I want to buy a house but how am I going to keep up with a house? Can I continue to drive as my symptoms get worse? How can I keep a job? Can I live by myself? All I can say right now is that I am asking the same questions I've had for years and I am hoping that this new set of specialists will have some answers and I'll find relief. Maybe God finally will say it's time for us to know. Maybe not."

"Courage doesn't always roar. Sometimes courage is the little voice at the end of the day that says, I'll try again tomorrow."-Mary Anne Radmacher

A Mama's Perspective

When Bri was 23, she asked me to find her a specialist; she wanted to try medications again. I wasn't aware that she was actually scared because her drinking was becoming a problem. I thought about her disorder, having the physical as well as psychological features, so I thought about a neuropsychiatrist this time around. I found Dr. PW about an hour and a half from our home and scheduled an appointment with him for Bri. He was awesome. He performed neurological tests that no other neurologist had done. He showed us how Bri had leftover "primitive (baby) reflexes" with extrapyramidal symptoms. He tapped between her eyes, the Glabellar Reflex, and she continued to blink with the tapping. He explained that this was not normal, normal people outgrow the blink response and after about two or three taps between the eyebrows, they quit blinking. He also stroked the palm of her hand and her fingers would curl around his pen, the Palmer Grasp Reflex. She also was displaying Nystagmus, where her eyes would flutter or jiggle when he had her follow his pen. There were two other reflexes that were abnormal. Dr. PW explained that there seemed to be some sort of damage to her frontal lobe as well as the Myoclonus Dystonia and that she would probably experience impulse control issues. (I would later learn that the Extrapyramidal Symptoms could be a result of psychoactive/psychotropic drugs and Bri had definitely been on them with the

Bipolar diagnosis. Was this why she was showing symptoms when her MRI's and CT scans had been normal but there seemed to be damage to the frontal lobe?) I also wonder now if these baby reflexes showed up after her year of taking the psychotropic medications for the Bipolar disorder. My dad during his neurological exam prior to her being medicated for Bipolar, didn't find anything.

Dr. PW started her on several different medications. Because she wasn't sleeping, she was becoming exhausted so he prescribed Modafinil. Bri loved it. She wanted to work at her job all day and all night on that medication. She also told him that she was still having nightmares and they were terrifying. He said that Minipress, a heart medication used off-label, was good at stopping nightmares so she started taking it and it really did help. She was still taking 50 mg of Trazodone for sleep but it really wasn't helping. He prescribed Flexeril as needed for the muscle spasms. He had her try Paxil for depression and Topamax for OCD. Topamax is used off-label to treat OCD and it works really well. However, some pharmacists and techs call it Dopa-max as it makes people lose some of their cognitive functioning. He also suggested a certain type of marijuana but Bri couldn't tolerate it as it made her paranoid. He had her get the one that is sedative (Indica) but it still really messed with her. Dr. PW also knew that alcohol could alleviate the myoclonic symptoms and they discussed her use of alcohol. He cautioned her to be very careful and that he would follow her very closely for its use.

21

A Mama's Perspective

A few months later, she was complaining of nerve pain so he prescribed Gabapentin. Within a month she was starting to have hallucinations, however, they were a lot like what she sees with the spirits and her abilities as a sensitive. She had had a frightening experience in her home and I thought that maybe she was being tormented by entities again so I had her smudge her house and I did a space clearing for her. She then started sleepwalking. The most frightening event was when she called me after sleep-walking where she had punched her hand through her basement window breaking the glass and cutting her hand. She bled all over her bed and all throughout the house not knowing anything about it until she woke up later horrified and called me over. It was a bloody mess. She was a server at Red Lobster at the time and she had noticed that she would have wet pants during her shift but didn't know why. She was obviously having urinary incontinence and this was a new symptom. Bri had an appointment scheduled for three months out for a medication checkup and we were going to talk to him about the new symptoms of hallucinations which were becoming more frequent and her loss of bladder control. In fact, I was starting to get frequent calls from her managers at work to come and pick her up because she wasn't doing well and they were very concerned about her.

One day in late Dec 2013, she had come over to our house for a brief visit and she decided that she was going to drive over to her aunt's house to watch the football game. About 20 minutes after she left, she came back to the house with a bloody nose and knee and she told me that she had wrecked her car and didn't remember anything about it. I was so confused, how could you not know anything about wrecking your car? She seemed stable enough so I went out to see where the accident had happened. I noticed her car, my mom's old Saab in our driveway dripping oil and other fluids. The engine compartment was smashed in and I honestly didn't have any idea how she had driven it home from about a 1/4 mile away at our neighbor's house. I left Bri to go down to the neighbor's house as the paramedics, police, and fire trucks had shown up. I told them that it had been my daughter and that she was up at our house shaken up, but nothing seemed broken. A few of the first responders went up to the house; I followed. They checked her out, the police came and told us that they weren't going to cite her because it looked like she had experienced a medical emergency. They told us that had she made it to the highway another mile down the road, based on their observations, they thought that her accident would have been deadly. Bri had not tried to correct or brake for anything. She went off of the road, flew over an irrigation ditch, took out the fence, went airborne for 20 feet, took out another fence, split an old wooden power pole in half, nicked an old cottonwood tree, and had just missed being impaled by a branch. The car had come to rest at the corner of the neighbor's garage at a brick planter. Somehow Bri got the car started when she came to and she drove herself to our house. The first responders wanted to take her to the hospital but I asked how bad she was and I declined when they said she was stable. I told them that she had a scheduled appointment in the morning with her neuropsychiatrist and that she had a neurological movement disorder but that none of her doctors had told her that she couldn't drive.

The next morning I drove her down to Dr. PW's for her appointment as I wanted to be in the appointment with her when she told him what was going on. I was suspicious that she was having a reaction to the Gabapentin as she hadn't been on it before. She had started it about three months earlier, then the hallucinations and sleepwalking started. After two months of taking the medication, Bri started having a loss of bladder control. I would realize later that she had been prescribed Neurontin (Gabapentin) years earlier, then was taken off of it after 10 days because of side effects. We told him about the hallucinations, the sleepwalking, and the loss of bladder control. He told us that these symptoms were indicative of a seizure disorder and that the bladder control issues were from absence seizures. With the total blackout, while driving her car, he was very concerned that she had been misdiagnosed with Myoclonus Dystonia and he wanted to rule out Progressive Myoclonic Epilepsy (PME) instead, which he told us was fatal.[11]

I pushed for him to consider that her new symptoms were side effects of the Gabapentin. He scheduled Bri for a three-day to seven-day stay at the Epileptic Monitoring Unit but it would be about three months away. At Bri's next follow-up appointment, Dr. PW told us that he was ill and was going to leave practice and move back to California. He didn't put us in touch with anyone to follow Bri, but he refilled all of her prescriptions to get her through to the EMU stay.

With Bri's black-out seizures becoming more frequent and continuing to worsen, she could not bathe alone. I, or her sister, would have to stay with her because she would pass out and not come out of the black-out seizure for over 10 minutes. Then she would have the postictal phase of the seizure where she would sleep for hours and be very confused. I decided that something needed to be done. I told Bri that I suspected that the Gabapentin was causing the new seizure activity and I wanted her to quit taking it which she did. Within a week she was doing much better and by two weeks she wasn't having any blackout seizures, hallucinations, sleepwalking episodes, or loss of bladder control. I had my answer but we still kept the appointment for the stay at the EMU just in case.

Bri's Perspective

I was so proud to purchase my very own home at the age of 19, and I had big plans for it. I thought this was a big deal! When my boyfriend said he couldn't take the night off of his lifeguard duty job, I realized he probably wasn't the right one for me. If he couldn't be happy for me in this, when would he ever be? After three years of dating, I drove down that night and broke it off with him. The house would be in a constant state of some project or another. With help from my mom and dad, I remodeled the place while going to school and working at a restaurant. I planned to flip it and use the money to invest in a nicer flipper and continue the cycle.

I loved my job as a server and bartender and I was good at it. I had the memory of an elephant and was never overwhelmed; I could easily remember orders without writing them down. I quickly became one of the lead servers, trainers, and bartenders. I could take on more tables than almost all of the other staff and loved the multitasking, fast-paced nature of the job. However, I started struggling with blackout episodes as well as a loss of bladder control and decided it was time to step back from work.

One day, I was on my way to my aunt's place with my dog when I remembered my dog jumping into the back of the car and onto the floorboard which was uncharacteristic of her. The next thing I remember is waking up at a neighbor's house, covered in blood, in my passenger seat, with all the airbags deployed. I checked on my dog who was unharmed, I crawled back into the driver's seat not knowing what had happened, started the car, and parked it back in my parent's driveway. I walked through the door and my mom said, "Bri, is everything ok?" I said, "I think I hit a pole". She ran over and saw me covered in blood. She drew me a bath, had my sister watch over me, and left to talk to the emergency responders. I had suffered only a sprained knee and a bloody nose while my car was severely damaged. I was extremely thankful my dog was unharmed. I'm guessing she was protected due to her sensing what was happening and diving onto the back seat floorboard. My little dog, Bean, had been with me for several years and she could always sense when things were about to happen. I also think my deceased grandma had been in the car with me to protect me that day. The neighbor who saw the accident asked how we were doing despite me being the only one in the car. He claimed he had seen two women in the car and told the emergency dispatch that there were two people in the car.

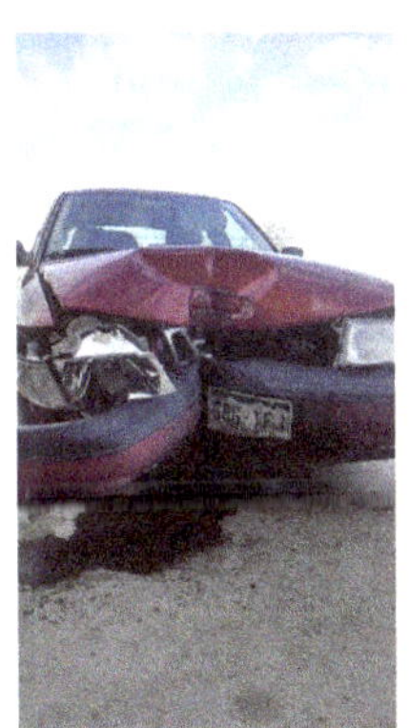

**Medication Side
Effect - Blackout
Crash**

22

A Mama's Perspective

Three months after her car accident, I took Bri to the hospital. I stayed with her while they got her settled in and applied the pads to her scalp for the three-day EEG test and neurological evaluation. Later in the afternoon, I was starting to worry about my dad who I hadn't heard from in recent days. Five years earlier, after my mom passed suddenly from a massive heart attack at 69 years old, dad had told my brother and me that he had a "Triple A" and to look it up. He was referring to an abdominal aortic aneurysm. He indicated that his was huge, over 6 cm. Being a doctor, he knew what the risks were for having a stent put in and he wasn't willing to risk it. He preferred living out his life despite knowing that when it ruptured, he'd probably have about 15 minutes before he died. This didn't sit well with my brother but I knew that my dad wanted to live life to the fullest, which he did for the next five years. He would take his boat out to Lake Powell and be gone for up to a week or he'd take his little camper somewhere without a cell phone to contact any-one. About seven days into his spontaneous adventures, my brother would start to get upset. I'd tell him to give dad another day or two and if he doesn't come home, I'll send out the search team. He always came home within 10 days. He was a pilot, so he had me fly with him every week. Having not heard from him in several days,

I started getting anxious. I hated to leave Bri but I really felt that something was off. Family friends checked on Bri, and one stayed with her. That eased my mind as I left to check on my Dad.

As I drove down the highway I noticed a sign with the name Monarch on it. I believe in synchronicities; my parents had paid a cremation service called Monarch for their cremations. This particular company would take their remains anywhere in the world and cremate them and ship them back to the US, or if they were in the US, they would provide the service here. My parents traveled a lot on their sailboat so they didn't want my brother and me having to deal with anything if they were to die. So, my first "clue" was seeing the Monarch sign. Next, I saw a hearse going down the highway; I was really starting to feel anxious. As I got closer to my dad's house, I passed a cemetery and I prepared myself to find that my dad had passed. I rang the doorbell and he didn't answer but his truck and toys were at the house. I used my key and called out to my dad. I found him deceased in his bed with a heating pad on his tummy.

The next few days were a whirlwind. I tried communicating with Bri's neurologists at the hospital to tell them that I was suspicious that she had been reacting to the Gabapentin. My husband had taken over being with Bri. Only one of the five neurologists half-heartedly agreed that it was the Gabapentin, because the tests were all normal. She was sent home after three days.

Bri's Perspective

I was scheduled for a three to seven-day EMU stay, as they tried to induce a seizure. What this looked like was being hooked up to an EEG 24/7, not being able to leave the hospital bed because of the seizure risk, and the doctors keeping me awake 23 hours of every 24-hour period. An hour after I was admitted, as the nurses started hooking me up, my mom said she had to go check on her dad. I was a little frustrated because I heard this statement from her almost every other weekend and we had JUST gotten to the hospital (which I didn't want to be at in the first place.) After she left, I wondered "what if he has passed?" She called me not long later, softly crying, to tell me that my grandpa had died. So I was now stuck, in a bed, hooked up to a machine, not able to sleep, and I was supposed to deal with this news? He was my role model growing up. His thirst for life and adventure was ingrained in me. I had always wanted to impress him. One of my favorite memories was the time in a hot spring that could get up to 115 degrees he casually sat down and I joined him. The water was so hot it took what seemed like forever to fully sit down. Each time anyone moved the water at all, it was like I was getting in all over again. Of course, once I felt like the badass I thought I was - he dunked his head under! So, of course, I followed suit.

The nurses were very sweet and all signed a card for me about my loss but I knew if I started crying I wouldn't be able to stop. I pushed that grief down along with so many other things I had to push down over the years. The EMU was painfully boring; 1 tried coloring and watching TV. A couple of my friends would spend some time with me. Eventually, they ended it and I was able to go home. Once again, a normal test. We would later learn that with Myoclonus Dystonia, imaging tests are normal unless there is another underlying condition like epilepsy or a tumor or an injury. Because my imaging tests and EEG's were all normal, a lot of the first neurologists and first movement disorder specialists missed that I had Myoclonus Dystonia. It was always bittersweet, having normal tests, yet not feeling well with no reason for my symptoms.

23

A Mama's Perspective

We took Bri home and she wasn't followed by another specialist for several years. She lived alone, continued to go to school and work full-time. At this point, I was so frustrated with specialists that I went into a funk and quit trying to help for a while. I was also hearing from my husband's side of the family, through my daughters, that I should just stop researching things, and taking Bri to different doctors; that I was just making things worse. This really upset me. I felt like I had very little support, and my husband's family saying I was causing problems was very hurtful. They didn't understand; I felt like they didn't really want to understand.

> *"It's interesting. People go to an animal shelter and pick a dog that's been kicked, beaten, and has lost a leg and an eye, and they'll take that dog home and give it love and support, but they don't do that with people."-Nikki Sixx*

We had also felt a loss of support through our church earlier. It seemed as if our church family grew fatigued when the diagnosis was never clear. Was it easier if a person was going to die? Then they could pray for comfort and peace. Or better yet, a person had something that had a cure and would be healed in due time, viola, prayers answered. But with a chronic condition, and a very rare one at that, it felt as if our church family had given up, unable to follow what was the latest news. It seemed that their prayers, along with ours, were not being answered; it was all very disconcerting.

I felt as if I had given up at this point. I hadn't of course, I was just frustrated and scared. I didn't want what was going on in our family to be the sole topic of conversation with our friends. I started isolating myself from friends so that I wouldn't always seem to be complaining. I also grieved the loss of my daughter's youth, when our friends would share how awesome their kiddos were doing. We were stuck on the spin cycle of a very rare and incurable disorder. Our daughter was doing her best to survive. My husband was also very tight-lipped and no one at his company knew what we were dealing with, and had been dealing with, for 13 years. My parents had both passed on, and I was feeling very alone.

Bri's Perspective

My mom wouldn't give up, despite what she might say, but I had. No answers, no solutions, just a world of pain. I knew my sister was feeling neglected because no matter how much I begged my mom to let it go, she wouldn't. I was angry at my extended family for blaming my mom for my illness. They had no idea what she gave up trying to help me. Their go-to was to place blame. Much like my mom, I had isolated; but unlike my mom, I had also given up.

24

A Mama's Perspective

We had decided to take a break from neurologists/movement disorder specialists but I was still very concerned for Bri and the amount of pain that she was dealing with daily. Bri had no pain medication, although it's efficacy in the past was questionable. I had reached out to Bri's prior hypnotherapist and asked him if he knew of any methods that might address Bri's pain. Hypnotherapy, surprisingly, had not helped her. I found this really perplexing because my dad had used hypnotherapy on my mom to help her have dental work, including crowns, without any anesthetics because she reacted to so many medications. My mom was also able to have minor surgeries under hypnosis. I told my friend that Bri was still dealing with a lot of pain, along with her other symptoms, and I wondered if there was a good therapist whom she could talk to. He suggested that Bri see Dr. JR who had treated 9/11 burn victims by using Mindfulness Meditation techniques. She had recently moved to Colorado from New York and had had great success with using Mindfulness Meditation to address pain.

Bri started going weekly but I could tell within just a few short months that this technique wasn't working. After about four months she quit seeing this therapist. We wouldn't figure out why hypnosis and Mindfulness Meditation seemed to fail with Bri until much later in her journey. Both therapies failed to bring any relief whatsoever and I was astonished. Years later we learned why, and started the process of finding out what therapies did work.

25

A Mama's Perspective

Bri had a boyfriend that she had known for years through our church. He had been the wonder boy that all of the parents wanted their daughters to marry. Well, appearance can be deceiving, and after a few months together they broke up. Bri had lent him money to buy a car to get to work because his car wasn't running. When they broke up, she didn't think that he would pay her back, but he did give her the money. She decided that she would treat herself to a trip and she booked one for the Dominican Republic. About ten days after she got back, she started getting ill with fevers, the shakes, nausea, vomiting, a temperature, sweating, insomnia, anxiety and some other symptoms. I didn't know what to make of it all. I suspected that she had picked up a bug while on vacation, but after three weeks of her being ill, I put the symptoms into an illness checker and it seemed possible that she contracted malaria.

Bri's Perspective

I had made a promise to myself that if this guy paid me back for the car, knowing how unlikely this would be, that I would treat myself to a solo vacation. When he paid me back in full, I went straight to a travel agent to help me. I was both excited and nervous as I was about to find out if I actually liked myself. Turns out, I did! I had a blast and met several amazing people. Although I had been drinking quite heavily before I went on the vacation, going alone, I knew I would have to control myself. So, I drank minimally. To this day I am thankful that I did because I remember the whole vacation, my great adventures, and the angels I met on my way home. I enjoyed making new friends that I still talk to today, meeting a couple of girls on a catamaran day cruise, getting bit up by mosquitos and sand fleas on a remote island. The most memorable experience was taking a day tour up the countryside of the Dominican Republic where I ended up jumping off of a waterfall into the "Fountain of Youth" and bathing in the "healing" mud.

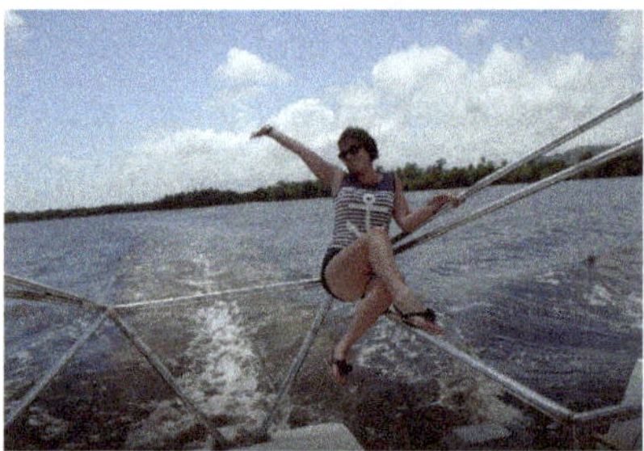

Boat Tour in the Dominican Republic

However, upon my return home I became ill and I reverted to drinking heavily. I realize now that when I am ill from something other than my disorder, my symptoms increase, and without medications or any alternatives to alleviate the symptoms, I revert to alcohol even when I'm ill. I've been so used to headaches and not feeling well that drinking's ill effects aren't a big deal. I usually feel like crap whether I drink or not.

A Mama's Perspective

The symptoms and onset of symptoms fit for malaria. There was an outbreak of malaria where she stayed on the island. I contacted the Centers for Disease Control (CDC) for advice on where to take her and how to get tested. Over the next several weeks, we visited several ER's. If testing wasn't done correctly, then the tests were not reliable according to the CDC. The ER doctors weren't sure about what was going on. Her dad and I eventually made an appointment for her with a travel illness doctor. He took her history and at one point he asked if she was abusing any substances. She replied that she wasn't and we believed her. He drew some blood work and I think he knew what was going on by the time he got the results but he didn't challenge her on the substance abuse issue. We didn't return for any follow up when he said that she didn't have malaria. I wished he told us what he had found, that she had extremely high blood alcohol levels, but he didn't. The Medical Power of Attorney for Bri that we had drawn up when she was 19 didn't seem to make any difference. Even with Bri's permission to share information with us, he still declined to go there. About 60 days into Bri's "illness", her elderly neighbor and her daughter called us in a panic. They said that Bri came to their house, walked in very confused, and asked weird questions. They always had an open door for Bri and her sweet little dog Beanie. My husband and I dropped everything and drove up to see what was going on. Bri was disheveled, confused, and incoherent. We put her in our truck and looked at each other knowing, but not wanting to say anything. We drove in silence back to our house; I cried silently the entire 30-minute drive. We got Bri settled into her old bedroom.

The next three days were absolutely terrifying. At one point, I smelled very sweet breath on Bri and I thought she was throwing off Ketones. I ran out to the 24-hour pharmacy and got some ketone strips to test her but they were normal. I asked Tara if she thought Bri was acting like she was drunk and she said, "Yes." I was absolutely in denial regarding my daughter's drinking. I don't know if it was the stigma of having an alcoholic daughter, or that I just couldn't believe that she had succumbed to her disorder's propensity for alcohol abuse. I know that I was desperately looking for answers in every direction except the one pointing to substance abuse. She was so anxious, sweaty, and delirious. I couldn't deal with it anymore so I scheduled an appointment to see her primary care physician regarding what she knew about Bri and her illness.

Well, I took my Medical Power of Attorney with me to the doctor's visit and I flat-out asked her what was going on. (She knew that Bri was trying to quit alcohol.) She said that they had been talking for several weeks, but instead of her telling me what was going on, she said to go to the ER immediately. I did as she said and took Bri to the closest ER. I was really scared at this point and I hadn't had any sleep for 72 hours. Dr. WC came in to assess Bri and I tried to explain to him that Bri had traveled outside of the country, and that she had a very rare and incurable neurological movement disorder called Myoclonus Dystonia. He was not impressed. He ordered blood work and we just weren't seeing eye to eye. I had asked him to call a doctor friend of mine to verify that Bri did indeed have a disorder and that she could experience extreme anxiety and panic disorders with it. Hours later he came in and told me that Bri was an alcoholic and that she had a blood alcohol level of 0.4! I knew that this level was extremely dangerous and could be deadly. However, he was anything but caring and I fell apart. I had to call my husband to come to the hospital as I was so angry that I could hardly see straight. My husband arrived about a half hour later and I went home. He talked with the ER doctor, then called a friend who had been in rehab. They were able to get Bri a bed that night and her dad drove her down for a 21-day stay. Bri agreed to go because she knew how mad we were at her. She was in withdrawal and felt like crap; she had no fight in her.

We weren't allowed to visit her for the first few days, but then we were required to attend therapy sessions twice a week. Bri was put on Lyrica and within days she was having absence seizures and loss of bladder control. I immediately called and told them that they had to take her off of it or she would start having blackout seizures. She was on it for a week, then quit, and stopped having problems. During therapy sessions, we were told that the success rate for rehab was about 12% for first timers and it got progressively worse each time they re-entered. This didn't sit well with me at all. The expense of the rehab at about $30,000 was outrageous for a best possible outcome of 12% remaining sober after leaving. I would later look into rehab centers and would find that they are not really regulated. They don't have to be successful. You just pay your money each time you go and they toss you out weeks to months later. They also admonished us to "cut Bri off" when she was in her addiction. I thought how brutal, she is dealing with a very rare and incurable neurological movement disorder without any effective therapy and you are suggesting that if she drinks, we toss her out onto the street so that she can be raped or worse? No way, not doing that. Our poor girl needed our help and support, not abandonment. I wouldn't want to walk a foot in her shoes, let alone deal with everything that she was trying so desperately to deal with.

Bri hadn't been on any medication for her disorder for a few years and she was panicked about leaving rehab without anything in place to control her disorder. We asked for special permission for her to leave rehab to see a movement disorder specialist. They agreed that we could take her out for the day. I had learned about the Dystonia Medical Research Foundation earlier and I had looked up doctors on their referral site. A certain doctor in northern Colorado said that she was a neurologist, psychiatrist, and a movement disorder specialist. I thought, oh my goodness, what a great trifecta of specialties. She should be very well versed in Myoclonus Dystonia, both the physical and psychological symptoms, and be prepared to deal with the alcohol abuse aspect too. Dr. TM even had the disorder listed as one of her areas of expertise.

Bri met with her and Dr. TM prescribed Cymbalta and Trazodone for sleep. She agreed with Bri's diagnosis of Myoclonus Dystonia. Bri was taken back to rehab and released on day 21 with her therapist telling us what a model patient she had been. He expected her to do very well with sobriety. She was also on prescription medications again. He gave us his phone number and said that we could call him anytime with concerns. Bri was to sign up for an outpatient rehab online that would cost her $1,700 out of pocket. She was responsible for her deductible. Bri came home and signed up for the online rehab.

Bri had started taking the Cymbalta; over the next two weeks, her mood declined. She also was starting to really have some bad myoclonic symptoms and was in a lot of pain. One night when she was supposed to be online attending her rehab she missed her class. She was thrown out and not able to attend anymore. They kept her $1,700 and I was absolutely furious. I spoke with the online coordinator and she said that I was an enabler. She explained they would not let Bri attend any more classes and that she wouldn't be receiving any portion of her money back. What a racket.

Bri's Perspective

"Today my forest is dark. The trees are sad and all the butterflies have broken wings."-Raine Cooper

I went to rehab knowing I was in over my head taking the doctors' drinking suggestions too far. I graduated 2nd of my rehab class; they told me I would be one of the few who made it. I wanted to make it, but I was doubtful. The drinking was my fault, this is what the therapists were telling me. Had I been prescribed benzos, or pain meds, and gotten addicted to them instead, I'd be innocent of my addiction. It would have been precipitated by my doctors prescribing them and they would have had some culpability in my addiction. My addiction would have come about because of prescribed medications, not because I was a loser with absolutely no control. Unfortunately, the root cause of my addiction to alcohol was blamed to be a defect in my character according to rehab and Alcoholics Anonymous, and not due to a painful, rare disorder that has alcohol abuse as a psychological feature. I would continue to be stigmatized as an alcoholic with a defective character for years, even by some family members.

A Mama's Perspective

Within two weeks, Bri had her first relapse and I called her therapist who had given me his phone number with instructions to call if we had concerns. When he answered and I explained what was going on, he chastised me and told me that I had no business contacting him. Wow! Unbelievable! I decided at that point that Bri would never go to another rehab and that there had to be other options.

26

A Mama's Perspective

Around this same time, we received the Explanation of Medical Benefits (EOMB) from the ER visit back in July 2016. The claim had been denied. Dr. WC had prejudicially labeled Bri as a "malingerer" or a faker! I was so angry that I could hardly see straight. He had no right to label her with such a stigmatizing and false label. This label would be so very damaging for Bri going forward trying to seek medical care. I dug into what the label meant for Bri and how in the world this malicious ER doctor thought that he could do such a thing. I contacted the Chief of Staff, Dr. PL, at NCMC in Northern Colorado and requested a meeting. He denied me a meeting. So, I began to send letters to his office to explain that a doctor can't label a patient because they are biased. If I could find a way to make Dr. WC face the music I would.

According to the National Library of Medicine, in order to label someone with malingering, five criteria need to be met: The first criteria is that the doctor labeling "malingerer" must be an expert at assigning this particular label, an expert in this field if you will. It is typically seen in Workman's Compensation claims. Secondly, the doctor must be in agreement with the patient's prior doctors that the patient is indeed a malingerer by using their medical history to prove a pattern. There are two other criteria but the last one is

92

critical, a "financial gain" for the patient. This ER doctor had not met, nor proved, any of these criteria. I explained this to the Chief of Staff. During one of only two phone calls that he would speak with me, he said that he didn't think anything would come of my daughter being labeled. I reminded him that having our insurance deny a $3,500 visit had already been harmful. I asked him if he would expunge her medical record of the stigmatizing label and he said that he couldn't and that I could "amend her records with information from her doctors."

I quickly set about amending the record with documents from her various doctors. The ladies in Medical Records definitely got an earful at just how unprofessional one of their ER doctors was. I made it a point to never have Bri, or any other family member, end up in that hospital. I would continue to write letters to the Chief of Staff over the next year informing him of just what damage this label was doing to my daughter. He didn't care.

I also contacted our insurance company and requested that we be given an advocate to help deal with the insurance issues we were having. I told our insurance company that they were never to pay North Colorado Medical Center (NCMC/Banner) for this visit if at any point they decided to do so. I learned that in Bri's medical records, the ER initially had given her the diagnosis of Anxiety for being admitted into the ER but Dr. WC changed it to malingering. The diagnosis of Anxiety would have been covered and the bill would have been paid. We had met our deductible. Our insurance company said that we could have the visit resubmitted with the primary diagnosis of Anxiety and they would cover it. I had the hospital resubmit it and about two years later I found out that our insurance had paid the hospital $1,500.

I can't fully describe the damage this doctor did to my girl, who wasn't a malingerer. I had never wanted to sue a doctor until this one. I did look into it, however, labeling a patient with malingering is not considered malpractice. I would later write a letter to the State of Colorado's Medical Board about the situation. They would look into it; then close the file. Bri had worked her butt off since she was 14, starting her burrito business and selling them before school. She had secured an apartment at age 17 and graduated high school with honors. Right before she turned 18 she moved out, was going to college, and working full-time. In college, she was receiving awards for ethics and attended many competitions. When she turned 19, she purchased her own home. We helped her remodel and update the property. She was no sloucher and she had never cried "oh poor pitiful me" in order to gain attention. She dealt with her disorder with a lot of strength, albeit, a lot of solitude, and introspection. In fact, the last thing that she wanted to do was to see a doctor or bring attention to herself! Despite everything she was going through internally and in secret, her mood seemed to be stable and consistent. Bri rarely, if ever, cried. I had only seen her cry a handful of times; in fact, I worried that she bottled everything up. She never lashed out with anger, or blame; she always suffered in silence. To be called a faker was devastating. Bri had never tried to garner attention, or profit financially from her disorder, which was a criteria for a diagnosis of malingering.

27

A Mama's Perspective

I was also starting to get a reputation. It was implied that Munchausen by Proxy might be causing my daughter's symptoms. Munchausen by Proxy is where a parent, or "proxy," makes up, or fabricates an illness or an injury in their child when they aren't really ill or injured. It is considered a mental illness in the caretaker making the claims. This really ticked me off. I felt like I was close to being labeled because of my efforts to find answers for my daughter, to be her best advocate. I think there are quite a few advocates who face this suspicion as well; it is unfair. Looking back, I realize that almost all of Bri's specialists were willing to give her a diagnosis, to put the diagnosis into her medical records, bill her insurance based on the diagnosis, prescribe her cocktails of medications whether or not they were effective or needed, and all while not really knowing if she truly had the diagnosis, or not! Instead of stating, "rule out," or, "at this time it may be," or whatever, almost all of them would give her a diagnosis. The worst diagnosis was Bipolar I Disorder, along with being medicated for it, although PNES was a close second.

The doctors we encountered along the way were nothing like my dad, he was old school. He would go to his colleagues with his difficult cases and they would give it their best-educated guesses until they had the correct answers. This was long before the Internet, which has been a game changer. Also, my dad was a General Practitioner licensed to treat patients from maternity, to birth and all the way through until death, along with treating emergencies and performing surgeries. The old-school doctors were well-versed in how the various body systems worked as a whole. In my opinion, specialists sometimes lose sight of how the body's systems are affecting each other, they are narrowly focused on their area of expertise. For example, in Bri's case, no one early on looked at how she had muscle cramps, muscle spasticity, twitches, tremors, jerks, nerve pain, and then the psychological symptoms of anxiety, depression, OCD, and panic disorder. It seemed as if they looked at the muscle symptoms (dystonia) separate from the myoclonus symptoms of twitches and jerking, and then these symptoms were considered separately from the various psychological symptoms. The psychological symptoms were separated from the physical symptoms, Occam's Razor was not being applied by her specialists to discover the overarching disorder that very much addressed each of her symptoms. It is kind of shocking, knowing that there are symptom checkers online that easily aid an individual, or a specialist, in weeding out the various diagnoses and then giving direction in diagnosing correctly. By searching Bri's various symptoms online, I was able to come up with Myoclonus Dystonia two years before Bri received the diagnosis in 2010; after many failures to diagnose her correctly by other specialists.

I am reminded by chronic illness sufferers, that our doctors work for us, and sometimes I think many of them need reminding of this fact too. I am generalizing, but it is from the frustration of two decades of very little heavy lifting by the specialists we saw. Instead of saying they didn't really know, they were quick to diagnose and prescribe and send us on our way. I would spend many, many, sleepless nights digging into professional journals and articles and research papers in order to find answers for my precious girl, when the specialists had failed to work for us to find the answers.

There is a meme that floats around the support groups for the chronic disorders, it goes like this: "Doctor to Patient: Don't confuse your Google search with my medical degree and expertise. Patient to Doctor: Don't confuse your medical degree with my 20 years of living with this disorder." I wish that more doctors would appreciate what a patient and their advocate are doing to help shed light on the situation and welcome their help and insight. I can't tell you how many people with chronic, and rare disorders, are very well versed in their disorder, even more so than their specialists at times, and yet are discounted.

The support groups we are involved in are a wealth of information that we just don't seem to receive from our specialists. For example, specialists still continue to say that Myoclonus Dystonia is not progressive. However, we have found through our support groups that in many cases Myoclonus Dystonia is progressive and its symptoms can also fluctuate with illness, temperature, stress, lack of sleep, physical exertion and other stimulation. Bri knows all of this to be true, she has experienced it. When it comes to digging into genetics, I'll admit, my eyes glaze over. Besides the rudimentary facts, it's all gibberish to me. I definitely felt unappreciated with many of Bri's specialists. Just because you don't have a medical degree doesn't mean that you are intellectually inferior. People can read content and understand complicated information and make decisions based on their educated understanding. It is really unfortunate that there seems to be an "us versus them" mentality in the medical profession these days. It's such a breath of fresh air when you end up with a specialist with whom you have a great partnership. It's wonderful to be able to share information and ideas and proceed forward together, as a team, and as it should be.

28

A Mama's Perspective

After being released from rehab and receiving her medication from the new specialist, Bri continued to worsen taking the Cymbalta over the next thirty days. She had never been on it before. About a month into taking it, she became suicidal. I contacted Dr. TM's office and spoke with her nurse. The nurse told me to call the suicide hotline. I was stunned. I had hoped that we could have Bri seen by the doctor as soon as possible.

The very next day a certified letter showed up for Bri from their office. Dr. TM wrote to Bri and told her that she was being discharged from the practice and that she had 15 days to find a new doctor. There was no explanation as to why Bri was being discharged from practice. I couldn't believe what we were reading. To be discharged and given 15 days to find a new specialist? This doctor wasn't going to wean my daughter off of the offending medication that was making her suicidal? You've got to be kidding me. I had to learn damn quick how to titrate Bri off of the Cymbalta, and in the meantime, I was frantically calling movement disorder specialists to secure an appointment for her as soon as possible. The earliest I could get an appointment for Bri was four months out and it was at the same clinic where she had been properly diagnosed but the doctor had caused so much trouble by suggesting that Bri could drink "if it helped."

I was suspicious that the label of malingerer that was now in her chart was responsible for this abrupt, and wholly unwarranted discharge, from the practice. We would later wonder if one of Bri's medications, previously prescribed by her neuropsychiatrist, Modafinal, could have been a reason for the abrupt discharge. It seems that this is a medication that can be abused and it is at least possible, that by requesting a refill, Bri made the doctor think she was abusing it.

With being maliciously labeled, and now discharged from her specialist's care abruptly, Bri in 2016 decided to sell her little house. We had loaned her the money to get new siding, new windows, a water heater, new electrical, and a furnace. She had purchased the 1927 little home for $35,000 and had lived there for five years putting $20,000 into it. We contacted our realtor and he suggested putting it on the market for $135,000, but before it hit the market, he had a ton of interest in it. It eventually sold for $149,000. Bri paid us back what she owed us and then decided that she would take her proceeds to move to San Antonio, TX. She didn't know a soul there. She wanted to live somewhere warm.

She leased a beautiful two-bedroom apartment that overlooked a gorgeous pool and a hillside of multimillion-dollar homes. I was excited for her and thought that she would get back on her feet, find a nice job and enjoy her life. She had a much different plan in mind; she really didn't care if she lived or died, and she just wanted to be in a beautiful place for what was going to happen next. She wasn't seeing any doctors and she wasn't on any medications. She had a huge distrust of doctors. To be honest, she had been mistreated by more than one. Things with specialists had gone from bad to worse so she was now on her own, and of course, her go-to of alcohol was the standard for self-medicating her disorder. In her new apartment, it was very easy to get alcohol with a delivery service. She had switched from drinking whiskey to drinking wine and she had started to binge drink instead of steadily drinking.

Bri's Perspective

I honestly don't know what I was thinking at the time. I had this soul-crushing feeling that I would die before I reached the age 28. I just had enough money for a beautiful place in San Antonio. As a teenager, I thought I was dying, and as an adult, there was no hope because the only remedy I knew to help me was alcohol, and that would destroy my life and the others around me. I just wanted to get away, and I could with my earnings from the sale of my home. So I did. I moved to a beautiful, top-floor apartment in San Antonio overlooking a beautiful hill and forest, as well as the pool. I stayed pretty unattached and went to AA daily. The attendees complained daily and it was depressing every time I went. I even had a sponsor who worked with me through the steps but it just didn't resonate with me. I didn't like their idea that if we fell off the wagon, that we had failed and had to start at the beginning even if someone had had decades of sobriety. Back to square one as a failure and lacking the character to remain sober. I tried to use this time to get sober and find meaning in life.

Every time I got sober, the pain and symptoms of my disorder would rear their ugly head. I would make sure to sober up a week before my family came to visit me in order to get past the obvious stages of withdrawal. I didn't want to disappoint them, but my life had been disappointing up to this point. I didn't know where to go, what to pursue, what to do.

However, even though I continued to binge drink, that wasn't my whole life. I love to explore. I would go tubing on the river or spelunking in San Antonio Cave systems and do other fun touristy things. I also tried to maintain a beautiful apartment and walked with my dog in the large park behind our apartments. I would get together with friends, ride motorcycles around the city, and try new restaurants along the way. I still tried to live a life keeping my drinking as close to my chest as I could.

29

A Mama's Perspective

Bri moved to San Antonio in January of 2017, driving herself down there with a U-haul in tow during a very nasty winter snowstorm. I had decided that I needed to cut some apron strings and let her be more independent, so I didn't offer to go with her. She made it to her new apartment and got things set up quickly. Her apartment was decorated beautifully and she had a great kitchen. She loves to cook, cooking is a meditative therapy for her, and I thought she was off to a good start.

However, the weeks started ticking by and Bri wasn't working. Then the three-day weekends started when I had no contact with her. She would be all bubbly texting and calling, but by Friday nights, she would be "off of the grid" until late Monday or Tuesday. I didn't know what was going on, exactly, but I had my suspicions. It was actually much worse than what I had told myself. Bri was drinking, binge drinking, and she would be detoxing throughout much of the weekends and into the week. In fact, she was ending up in the local ERs trying to detox. Even though I am listed as ICE (In Case of Emergency) in her phone, I never received a call from the hospital to let me know that she was there, alone.

By April things had taken a real turn for the worse and her dad and I decided that we needed to go down for a visit. Before we could get there, Bri would experience a near-death situation in which she died for eight minutes. Her dad and I arrived the next day and found our daughter very confused and vulnerable. She began to share with me what she had experienced. I knew right away that she had had what is known as a near-death experience. My grandmother had three, a friend from church had shared his near-death experience with me, and my mom over the years had introduced me to the phenomenon by giving me various books to read like Bettie J. Eddie's *"Embraced by the Light"* and others. I sat in awe as Bri told me what happened. It was the most fantastical and beautiful experience I had ever heard of. She has written a book about her experience called, *"White Flame."*

Bri was having an extremely hard time understanding what had just happened to her and she was very unsettled. I was fascinated with her every detail no matter how incredible they sounded. From what I had read about the near-death experience phenomenon previously, I was overjoyed that her life would be unfolding in miraculous ways. Maybe God had set her on a new path. Bri shared details that I had never heard of before like the dark, comforting, velvety void. I looked it up, and, sure enough, other near-death experiencers had nearly identical experiences with the void. Bri shared things that I had read about that were being theorized at the time, like time isn't linear, or the events she experienced on the other side might have all happened simultaneously. She would share each event in her NDE in a linear fashion while sharing her experience with others back on earth. Bri also saw binary code in her tunnel. There were also aspects of her experience that she just couldn't put into words. Many people who have near-death experiences have this quality of not being able to express what they experienced; it's just beyond words, ineffable. [12]

When I took Bri out for lunch, she sat next to the wall patting it with her hands. I asked her why; she replied that the walls were "just too solid." On the other side, she was able to merge with whatever she wanted to merge with; everything, including Bri, was pure energy. Here on earth, everything was just too solid. It creeped her out. I spent a week with her reassuring her that what she had experienced was very real, that my grandma and a friend had also shared their stories. I told her I had read several books about the phenomenon. I would continue to read up on it and share the information with her. I found out that life might not be as easy as I thought it would be after such an experience. The integration of a near-death experience isn't always as straightforward and rosy as I thought. In fact, people come back to find that their perceptions of the world are very different than from before their experiences. There are divorces, loss of friendships, changes in personalities, changes in life purposes and careers, and a multitude of other dramatic shifts. This would be the case for Bri as well.

I spent a week with her and thought that she was stable. Her sister came down for the next week to stay with her. After Tara left, it seemed like Bri might do okay. It was interesting that after her NDE, her symptoms of Myoclonus Dystonia seemed to disappear and she wasn't drinking anymore. I had read about cases of severe illnesses being completely healed during an NDE. I held my breath hoping that Bri too had been cured from her very rare neurological movement disorder and I started thanking God every night for curing her.

Several months went by and nothing seemed out of the ordinary, nothing frightening at least. Bri was communicating and not disappearing for several days at a time, although she still hadn't found work. She still had plenty of money; I encouraged her to find her passion. What I didn't realize is that Bri had not returned fully to this world. She was really struggling to know what was real and what wasn't. Near-death experiencers will tell you that they long to be Home, on the other side, and this is what Bri was feeling, she wanted to go Home. We visited her on several occasions during the next several months; she seemed very vulnerable and lost, but she wouldn't come home to Colorado.

30

A Mama's Perspective

During the summer of 2017, I found out that she was drinking again; her disorder's symptoms were coming back. I started my research regarding alternative therapies for alcohol abuse and found The Sinclair Method (Sinclairmethod.org). It is where you take a medication called Naltrexone about an hour before you expect to drink alcohol and it disrupts the pleasure centers in the brain so that, over time, your consumption of alcohol is reduced, even discontinued in some people. I thought that with this method, Bri might actually be able to have a drink once in a while socially. I thought that it would be nice to be "normal" as she had suffered from social isolation over the years. I still wasn't understanding how different an individual's brain is with Myoclonus Dystonia and how really dangerous it is for them to even drink one drink; but at this point, I thought that if it stopped her from drinking a second, third, or fourth drink, that it would have done its job. I asked Bri if she wanted to give it a try and she agreed.

I found a doctor who could prescribe the Naltrexone. When we went to dinner, she took her pill and ordered a drink. She barely drank it. Then she thought she'd try a beer but I was really reluctant and worried about her trying another drink. She ordered a beer but didn't touch it. I thought, oh my goodness, this stuff is a miracle!

Well, this would be short-lived. Bri didn't drink to be social, she drank to alleviate her Myoclonus Dystonia symptoms. When they hit, she didn't care to take the Naltrexone and wait an hour in order to drink. She wanted immediate relief.

I had really miscalculated how the Naltrexone would work for her. I didn't understand the severe nature of her abuse and how her brain is wired very differently. Alcohol abuse in Myoclonus Dystonia is still not well understood. I was treating her alcohol abuse as if it were the typical type of alcohol abuse. It is actually quite different, while it has many of the same mechanisms involved, it has the added twist of alcohol alleviating physically painful symptoms. With the complications of OCD and compulsivity, and not being able to stop drinking once they've started, even drinking one drink can set off a cascade of unwanted disasters.

31

A Mama's Perspective

On October 12, 2017 I got the worst phone call of my life. A neighbor of Bri's called me and told me that he had found her unresponsive in her apartment, that she was seizing, and that he had called an ambulance. It had taken the ambulance over 20 minutes to get to her. He didn't know where they had taken her. I immediately told my husband and we found a flight down as soon as we could. It was a two-day drive and the first time we could fly was also two days away, there just wasn't an option to get to her any sooner. I was having difficulty locating her, what hospital they had taken her to. I had learned from her monthly ER visits, earlier in the year, that no one would call me to tell me that she was in their hospitals. This time was no different. I also had to scramble to find care for her little Papillon, Bean. Bri had been taking her to a dog care center and I had their number. I called them and explained our situation. They were able to send a vet over to the apartment to take Bean for an extended stay at their facility. At least I didn't have to worry about her little dog, who also had seizures and needed care, she would be well taken care of until I could pick her up.

Bri was in the ICU and in a coma at a hospital just down the street from her apartment. We were told immediately upon our arrival that she wasn't expected to live! Her doctors told us that her sodium level, at 115, was "incompatible with life." Her dad and I were basically on a death watch. Time seemed to go very slowly for the

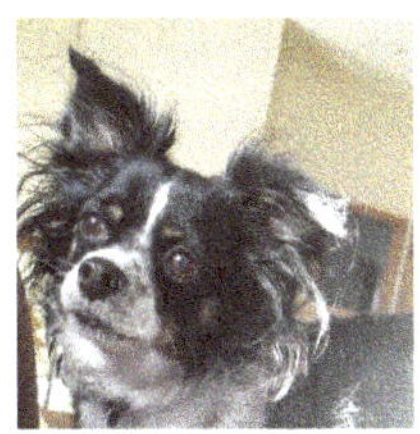

Ily Bean

next few days, as we waited for any change. Bri looked like the sweetest little angel, just sleeping peacefully in the bed, not a movement nor a sound. We were told by her doctors that she needed to be moved to another hospital for insurance reasons. We signed the paperwork to have her transferred but I wasn't too happy about it. We found out later that there was no need to transfer her but they did.

She was still in a coma going on four days. On the 15th, early in the afternoon, Bri abruptly woke up, and said that she was hungry. Her nurses rushed in and called her doctor. They discussed whether or not Bri could have something to eat and she requested a bagel. They told her dad and me, "Just watch her carefully and don't let her choke." Her doctor had spoken to us over the phone and she said that they would be moving Bri down to another floor for three days of observation before releasing her. Instead, a short six hours later she was being released into our care.

Bri had ended up with a low sodium level when she became dehydrated from vomiting for several days from a combination of an illness and detoxing from weeks of heavy drinking. She ended up in an alcohol withdrawal seizure and a coma from having a very low sodium level. Even her doctor at the hospital told us over the phone that she hadn't expected Bri to make it out alive. Curious then as to why she was sent home so abruptly, no one gave us an answer as to why just 6 hours earlier she was in a coma and now she was being sent home. I should have put my foot down, but I was overjoyed that she was coming home and she was alive.

We took Bri back to her apartment. My husband had to return to work the next day, so he flew back home. The hospital hadn't given us any instructions as to what to watch for. At least in Colorado, after an ER visit, we were given detailed instructions of when to reach out to her doctors, or when to come back to the ER. Instead, we weren't given anything. I was still confused as to why we had been told that Bri would be staying another three days, or so, for observation only to be released hours later. I wasn't too happy but my girl was alive so I was very thankful for that.

The first day back at her apartment went okay. She was very sleepy so I just let her sleep and I checked on her often. The next day, I noticed that she was having extreme difficulty walking. She would turn herself sideways, and kind of rock herself to get a leg moving. It was very weird and disconcerting. I also noticed that her speech was funny, she was slurring. We had been told verbally that she might still experience some detoxing symptoms and that we should watch for them and take her to an ER if concerned. With her inability to walk, kind of a spread eagle shuffle, walking sideways, huge lunging steps, and her speech difficulties, I took her to an ER. I explained what had transpired over the last week, and they gave her IV fluids and sent us home. By this time I had Googled her newest symptoms and found out that she had ataxia. This was very disconcerting and frightening.[13]

Another day passed; she soon started talking non-stop in a breathy and questioning voice. When I say nonstop talking, she just wouldn't stop talking and none of what she was saying was important. I Googled these new symptoms and found out that it is called Logorrhea or loquacity (talkativeness.) I took her to another ER, as the first one had been very disappointing. The ER doctor witnessed her ataxia but it wasn't a big deal to him. He gave her IV fluids, and again we were sent home without instructions. By this time, I had had enough of the hospital system in San Antonio. My husband got a flight for Bri to fly home to Colorado, where I could access better care for her from the comfort of our home. I put Bri on the plane, and had a flight attendant closely watching Bri until her dad picked her up. I picked up Bean, we packed a few things, and left for Colorado the next day in Bri's car.

Bri's Perspective

On one of my binges, I was determined to get sober AGAIN and quit cold turkey. I'm not sure how long this binge lasted, but I remember throwing up any water I tried to drink. I threw up in trash bags determined to empty them in the bathtubs as there was nothing solid in it. I had done it before. The last thing I remember is my legs getting cramps so bad that I was unable to release them. I next thing I remember, I woke up in the Intensive Care Unit feeling extremely hungry. I was once again filled with rage that I didn't just die that day. Many years later, I regret how I reacted to my neighbor who found me. I wasn't thankful; I was quite bitter towards him. I eventually apologized years later, but for someone who never took things out on other people, it was a painful and rare exception that I treated him without gratitude. I basically went to San Antonio to live until I died and when I came out of the coma still alive with no more answers than I went into it, I was not happy. I was almost free in my mind, but instead I was back to working my butt off to get to some state of normalcy again. After the coma, there were some brain damage issues that I needed some time and therapy to get through. The next few months are better explained by my mom, who again, never gave up on me.

A Mama's Perspective

When I got Bri back to Colorado, Bri didn't have a primary care physician and neither did I, so I took her to a local urgent care. I poured my heart out to the Physician Assistant who took a look at Bri. I explained as concisely as I could Bri's history with doctors, her rare disorder, her alcoholism and now her neurological symptoms after being in a coma from an alcohol withdrawal gone very bad. I begged for any kind of help we could get. The PA left the room for what seemed like an eternity, and when he returned he had the phone number of a neurologist who was willing to see Bri the very next day. I was speechless and very thankful.

Bri saw Dr. SF the next day and she was amazing. She knew about Myoclonus Dystonia and the effects of alcohol and that many sufferers become alcoholics. She told Bri that she would never judge her for her alcohol issues and that she should figure out how to abstain. She wouldn't be able to follow Bri for her disorder, she was more of a traumatic brain disorder neurologist and seizure specialist. However, she was able to set Bri up with Physical Therapy for the next three months. Bri worked very hard to get back on her feet, literally and figuratively. Her seizure and coma had left Bri with an infarction, or a stroke, in her HPA axis and it was going to be difficult to come back from that. Bri worked with a fierce determination and over the next three months she regained her ability to walk, although not very steadily. She had also quit talking so much, thank goodness. She decided that she was ready to go back to work so her dad hired her to write proposals and run the marketing department in the construction company that he ran. Bri excelled at her new position and things seemed to be looking up. She lived with us during her recovery.

32

A Mama's Perspective

With the TBI/infarction of her HPA axis in her brain, she had quickly put on 60 pounds in 60 days without explanation. I had Bri see an endocrinologist for the rapid weight gain, she wasn't on any medications so it wasn't coming from a side effect of a medication. She was eating an enormous amount of food though, she was just ravenous. Along with the three months of PT, Bri designed her own program for eating well and losing weight. She loves to cook so she came up with the most beautiful meals that were visually pleasing and very satiating. She lost 60 pounds over the next year.[14] Along with her weight loss and skills at proposal writing, she decided that it was time to become independent again. She had lived with us for a year since her coma and she was getting restless.

A recruiter found her and had a fantastic company in Atlanta, GA that was interested in Bri for proposal writing. After a few Zoom interviews, Bri flew down to Atlanta and had an interview and was hired. She came back home, put in her resignation, started packing and she was off to Atlanta. This time her dad and I decided to help her move. We had never been to Atlanta and she was moving downtown so that she could walk to work and all of the restaurants and shops. She had leased a beautiful, but small, apartment right across from all of the cool attractions in downtown

Atlanta. She was definitely going to be in her element, the downtown hustle and bustle of a big city. We were very excited for her. She hadn't had any alcohol in over a year, her Myoclonus Dystonia symptoms were in remission, she had lost all of the excess weight and she seemed ready to set the world on fire.

Everything was going very well, she was making new friends, enjoying exploring Atlanta and the surrounding areas, and she was loving her new job and apartment. Bean was adjusting well to apartment life. Then, in January 2020, Bri called us and asked if she could come home for a visit. We immediately said, "Yes." She had something she wanted to tell us. She arrived home in late January, told us that she had found a small lump on her thigh, and that she had seen a doctor. This particular doctor was a primary care doctor but had also done a residency in oncology. This doctor had sent Bri for a biopsy suspecting it was cancer. It was indeed cancer, a Soft Tissue Sarcoma, a rare cancer. At the time, I didn't realize just how unsettled Bri was about this new medical condition. She was scared and she had good reason to be. Her dad's side of the family has a saying that, "If cancer doesn't kill you when you're young, then you"ll live to a ripe old age where it will get you." My husband's family is riddled with different forms of cancer, some of his close relatives have died from cancer in their early 40's. There is a genetic condition called Li-Fraumeni Syndrome where different cancers are found in the different generations of a family with some dying quite young. I highly suspect that this is what my husband's family is dealing with, however, we haven't had the genetic tests done yet.

We tried to comfort Bri as much as we could and let her know that she had our support; whatever she needed she just had to tell us. We put her on the plane back home and I started Googling everything I could about Soft Tissue Sarcomas and the various doctors she was seeing. By early February, Bri was seeing a Sarcoma specialist. This is exactly who I wanted her to be seeing. Sarcomas are quite different from other cancers and a person really should see a Sarcoma specialist over a regular oncologist. I was happy that this particular specialist was out of Emory University Hospital, a very reputable teaching hospital. I felt that she was in good hands. She was put on a daily oral chemotherapy drug called Methotrexate and a daily oral therapeutic drug specifically for her type of sarcoma, Pazopanib, in order to halt the tumor's growth and possibly shrink it while she waited for surgery to remove the tumor. I looked up Pazopanib and its uses and I was horrified to see that it is used in end stage kidney cancer, however, it was being used for Bri with her soft tissue sarcoma. Bri had to tell her work what was going on and they immediately sent her home to work remotely. It wouldn't be long before everyone was sent home to work remotely because of the global pandemic.

Bri's apartment was nice but it was also dark, being on the first floor and looking out into the courtyard of a four-sided several-story building. It was also small and because of Covid, the common areas of the gym, pool, lounging areas and meeting rooms had all been shut down, so there was no contact with her neighbors and nowhere to go for a change of scenery. Downtown Atlanta had been shuttered. Except for getting the occasional groceries, Bri was isolated and without friends, or family, all while enduring a very scary and uncertain time dealing with a frightening cancer and taking medications that were making her ill. Because of Covid, the hospitals weren't scheduling any surgeries so Bri had no idea how long she'd have to wait to have her tumor excised. Knowing her dad's family history of various cancers, this had to be terrifying, living with this cancer in her body. This all just added to her anxiety and she began to drink again. Finally, on May 14, 2020, she had her tumor removed and the lab report was good news, all the margins were clear. She would need to schedule a follow-up for 6 months to check for any metastasis. Soft Tissue Sarcomas, especially when they have originated in the arm or the leg, have a bad habit of metastasizing to the lungs or liver, so people need to be followed very closely for many years later to catch metastases very early.

33

A Mama's Perspective

Bri continued to work remotely and even while being isolated, she somehow came down with Covid in July 2020. She completed her cancer therapies but they had left her immune Is system very weak and vulnerable. Bri wasn't feeling better and she ended up with what they are calling Long Haul Covid. By September 2020 she had lost her job. A lot of people were being laid off from her company, an international architectural firm. She tried to look for work but it was pointless, everyone was in the same boat. We told her to come home, that she had a safe place to land.

One night I was talking to her on the phone and she suddenly said that her jaw was locked in an open position and she started talking funny. I gave her some reassurance and said to let me know how she was doing in an hour or so. She called back and was in considerable pain. I sent her to the nearest urgent care facility, just down the street from her apartment, and the doctor there gave her some medication but said to go to the ER if things didn't improve soon. She ended up in the ER. She waited 12 hours; they took a look at her but by this time she was having symptoms of Myoclonus Dystonia and they were concerned about those. She was trying to tell them that it was her jaw, that she was having a lot of pain, and that the other symptoms were not the reason for her visit. Finally a facial surgeon came in to see her and was shocked that Bri hadn't been treated yet, knowing what kind of pain Bri was in. Bri had a fully dislocated jaw! The surgeon told Bri that she was going to put it back into place but that it was really going to hurt, and it did, but Bri was a trooper. She was given a prescription for Baclofen and told not to yawn or open her mouth too wide for several weeks.

34

A Mama's Perspective

In October 2020 Her dad and I went down and helped her pack up to move back to Colorado. Her dad kept saying that this was the last time he would help her move. Ha! I also noticed during our visit that Bri was having really bad tremors. I suspected that she was reacting to the Baclofen that was prescribed after her total jaw dislocation. I was very concerned that taking this particular medication might leave her with Tardive Dyskinesia, as Bri seems to always get the weirdest, and rarest side effects to medications. I certainly didn't want this particular disorder to set in and complicate matters. My mom was like this, she couldn't take much of any medication without suffering the side effects, even the rarer ones. In fact, one time, my dad was so perplexed by her reactivity to medications that he talked with her doctor and they decided to try a placebo experiment on her. Maybe not ethical but they had to know. She had been reacting to a certain medication and fainting which was a really rare side effect to the medication, so her doctor and my dad went to their pharmacist and had him create a pill that looked just like the prescription pill she was taking. She stopped fainting and they had their answer and she was given another prescription that she didn't react to. This is also why she was taught self-hypnosis, in order to avoid medications.

Bri's Perspective

After dealing with the after-effects of San Antonio, I moved home and worked really hard to get back to "normal." I pushed myself with PT and returned to the corporate world. I was told it was time that I start looking elsewhere, because my dad was supposed to retire and the owners might not need me. I was recruited from an international architectural firm in Atlanta. I was so excited; when I was in fifth grade I wanted to be an architect, but found out how long that process actually was, so this was the next best thing.

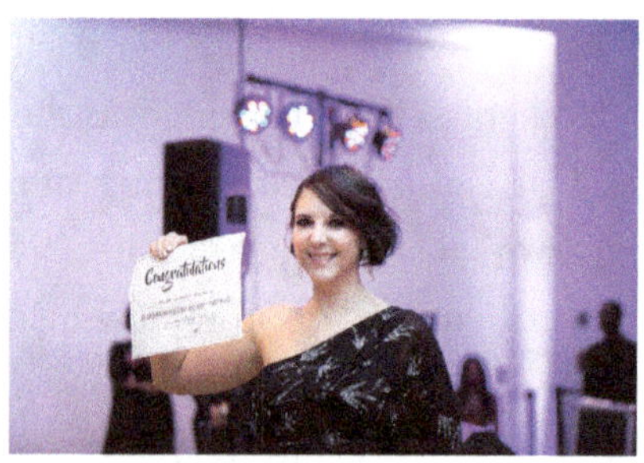

Winning the raffle at the company Christmas party

I had lost the 60 pounds I gained right after my coma. I lived and worked in downtown Atlanta; I had wonderful neighbors. I loved life. I enjoyed working with all of my coworkers in a 50-story building in the heart of downtown that was within walking distance. My apartment was next to Centennial Olympic Park and I walked my dog there every day. My apartment was stunning, less than 2-years old. I was the first person in my unit. They had an in-house dog wash and a mail concierge. There were water fountains outside my window and a rooftop pool that overlooked the World of Coca-Cola, the Civil Rights Museum, and the Aquarium. I made my first group of real friends since high school and we would get together for cooking parties, game nights, and dance our hearts out at the rooftop lounge. I had friends of all backgrounds, races, religions, and country origins. I was in heaven!

I would often walk to midtown to explore the hip new restaurants and walk back, about a 3-mile round trip. I would use the weekends to take my car to travel throughout other parts of the East

Coast. One of my favorite trips was a scenic railroad trip from Blue Ridge, Georgia to just across the Tennessee border. I would explore anything from state parks like Stone Mountain, nature preserves hidden within the city, cave systems, lakes, and waterfalls. During the week, I would work with amazing professionals compiling proposals together for anything from our local colleges to huge master plans in Saudi Arabia. It felt like I was living my best life.

Just a couple of months into living in Atlanta, I found a lump on my leg that wouldn't go away so I got in to see the doctor and was diagnosed pretty quickly. I once again fought to get through this as I fought to get through every hurdle in my life thus far. I refused to let it bug me and before we could schedule surgery — the world shut down. Covid happened; I was the first to be sent home from our office. I managed to deal with the diagnosis and treatment pretty well. The two weeks at home in my apartment turned into 4, which turned into "indefinitely". The park by my house was closed due to riots and all the amenities in my apartment were closed. What used to be a beautiful downtown apartment retreat, became my prison. The only place that was open was, ironically, the liquor store.

I acquired Covid around the fourth of July. Most of my neighbors ignored the restrictions and were going looney from solitary confinement as well. We ended up having a get-together, a BBQ. Two of us came down with covid right after. I didn't recover for quite a while. As my physical and mental health deteriorated, and I lost my dream job, I moved back to Colorado . . . again.

35

A Mama's Perspective

Bri moved home and we told her to get her health in order. We knew that she had started to drink again because her disorder's symptoms were coming back and we were monitoring it. In March of 2021, a recruiter contacted her for a position as a proposal writer for a very large construction company in south Denver. Bri hadn't been looking for work but she was feeling a little better and she just couldn't sit still. With her brain always in excitement mode and in a "go-go" state, she decided to accept the job offer and started commuting about an hour and a half each way a couple of days a week. Bri also started looking for apartments closer to her new job.

About a month into her new job, she started feeling funny and she ended up passing out at work. Right before she blacked out, she mentioned that she had a disorder and to please not call an ambulance, that she would be alright. However, her coworkers called an ambulance and she was taken to the ER. By the end of the week, she had lost her new job. She had not been drinking. She needed to have her sarcoma follow-up and without insurance, the MRI would have been very expensive, along with the specialist's appointment, and if they found anything, she was without insurance. Her dad needed her help and quickly hired her back at his company to work in marketing and proposal writing so that she could have insurance.

Over the next few months, Bri decided to go live with a friend. We weren't too happy about this. Bri was starting to get frantic because her Myoclonus Dystonia symptoms were returning and she wasn't on any medications. She started to increase her alcohol intake and desperately wanted to hide this from us so she started self-medicating with alcohol. She ended up binge drinking on several occasions; her dad was furious with her as she had missed a few Mondays at work. He told her that he would not cover for her.

By August of 2021, Bri was in need of safely withdrawing from alcohol and she actually requested time off to go into rehab. I wasn't too excited with this prospect as the first rehab had been a complete failure and the money involved was outrageous. The percentage for success at remaining sober was dismal. However, Bri was the one who requested rehab so we took her for a 28-day stay.

This rehab was different. They had alternatives to Alcoholics Anonymous. This was good news because Bri didn't resonate with AA. She was also getting counseling that was quite different from the first rehab stay and it seemed to be resonating with her. On the 14th day of a 28-day approved stay, we got a call from Bri saying that the facility had an outbreak of Covid and everyone was being sent home. I immediately drove 6 hours over to the front range to pick her up and bring her back to Montrose to stay with me. She stayed for two weeks, then went back over to the front range to go back to work. My husband had been living in the northern Colorado area during the week to work, and coming home to Montrose for the weekends, so he allowed Bri to move in with him.

36

A Mama's Perspective

During Bri's stay in rehab in August, I started following the Facebook support group Myoclonus Dystonia and another Dystonia group. I had seen a beautiful young woman named Meg who was asking about her hairstyle for her upcoming second Deep Brain Stimulation surgery. She had a blonde pixie and she was drop-dead gorgeous. I reached out to her to ask her about the surgery; she suggested that I call her so that we could talk. I found out that she was having a second DBS surgery after a device failure. Her neuro-stimulator unit and leads had been taken out and she had spent months in a rehab learning to walk again. She asked me to send her some videos of my daughter showing her symptoms and said that she would show her neurologist. What I didn't realize is that she meant that she was going to show her neurologist immediately upon receiving the videos; she was in the hospital recovering from her second DBS surgery when she showed him! Unbelievable! We call Meg our Earth DBS Angel and I credit her for saving Bri's life.

Bri's Perspective

I didn't know where else to go, so back to rehab it was. However, once sober for 10 days, I noticed twitching starting to return and wondered how bad it was going to get. About 14 days into my stay, and actually being excited to be learning some helpful tricks, we had a Covid outbreak. I went home. I finished out my time in Montrose with my mom. I was grateful to be with her, as the Myoclonus Dystonia came back in full force, and then some. I was also grateful for the time I had left, as I was trying to figure out who to see and what to do about the alcohol issues and the Myoclonus Dystonia symptoms. I thought it was going to be a long and painful journey forward. That is until my mom told me about Meg – who I now call my angel.

A Mama's Perspective

Meg called me a few days later and said to contact her neurologist, Dr. BA immediately, that he wanted to see Bri as soon as possible. I had Bri reach out to Dr. BA, a pediatric neurologist who specializes in Myoclonus Dystonia and Deep Brain Stimulation surgery, to make an appointment. He could see her the next week, but Bri needed to get time off from work so they scheduled her appointment for Friday, October 29, 2021. Bri flew out to Kansas City on her own and saw Dr. BA at 3 pm. She was having non-stop tremors and she had been losing her ability to walk over the last few months. Her symptoms were obvious and severe. Dr. BA spent about an hour with her going through her history and symptoms. He had already seen various videos of her symptoms. He then asked Bri why it had "been so long" and why no one had offered DBS to her. He called his neurosurgical team and sent Bri over immediately to get the DBS consult. Bri ecstatically called her dad and me and told us the fantastic news, she was being pre-approved for DBS surgery! I had not anticipated such good news. I was thinking that he would put her on some more medications for up to six months and then re-evaluate her. Nope. He did ask her to try Zonisamide as this was supposed to be a very effective medication but he also warned her about cognitive side effects and said to stop the medication if she felt changes. Sure enough, within two weeks, she was feeling off. So, on to DBS surgery.[15]

When Bri got home and started telling us all about her appointment and that she was being approved for surgery and that her surgery was being expedited, we could see her dad's face. His understanding now of the gravity of her situation hit him like a ton of bricks. He was kind of shell-shocked at the news. This was very serious. The last time that he had been to a specialist's appointment was years earlier when he had attended the one where Bri was told that she had Psychogenic Non-Epileptic Seizures and that it was basically "all in her head." Now her dad was being told that she indeed had a very rare neurological disorder, that medications had failed her, and her only real option at having a life was to implant electrical leads into her brain and zap her brain into submission with electrical stimulation. Dr. BA wanted to do surgery in November but Bri was required to have three surgeries over a three-week period so she would need to get time off of work. The soonest the surgeon was available was February 3, 2022. My husband found us a cute little Airbnb in a quiet neighborhood close to the hospital for the three-week stay.

37

A Mama's Perspective

About ten days before we were to leave for Bri's life saving surgery, I was still over in Montrose when Bri was having terrible symptoms and decided to drink heavily. I wasn't planning on leaving home for another eight days or so, but she was having a very bad withdrawal. I was so very angry with her. When I got over to her, I was so mad, I was yelling at her and telling her that she might have blown her only chance at having surgery. I was worried that Bri, being in withdrawal, might result in her surgery being canceled. I had to call Meg for her to walk me back from the edge of the cliff of anger and frustration. Meg and her family, too, have had to deal with the horrific psychological features of the disorder, especially the alcohol abuse feature. The term "'feature" has such a benign ring to it. Instead, it is the nastiest and scariest feature of the disorder, in my opinion. Meg did a fantastic job and calmed me down so that I could support my daughter in one of the most important times of her life. Bri had a few difficult days ahead but she came around and we left for Kansas City. Her dad flew out for her first operation.

Bri's Perspective

I had spoken with Meg and was told to get in touch with Dr. BA. He was able to see me the following week which blew my mind as it seemed like every specialist in the 20 years prior had a months long waiting list. I got the first trip that work would allow me to take. I saw him at the end of the month.

I made this trip without any preconceived notions. I was not excited because of my history with doctors and the medical field, and I understood that it might be a complete bust. I really went in trying to be non-judgemental and unpresuming. I ended up at a beautiful hotel and tried really hard to remain sober and on task. It really tested my resolve as there were free drinks until 10 at the bar in the lobby that night. I stayed sober and made it to my appointment in a full Myoclonic and Dystonic episode which has never happened in front of a doctor before… it was a good start.

After observing me not being able to sit still in the chair, Dr. BA felt terrible that no one had offered DBS before. He immediately sent me to the surgeon's office, at 4 pm on a Friday, to talk about DBS. Meg and her fiance drove me there and Meg was with me for both appointments. While Dr. BA wanted to do the surgery immediately, I wouldn't get the scheduling call for another week.

My dog had been killed earlier that year and I was thinking it was time to find a new one after watching my friends' dogs. I saw an adoption event on Saturday, November 6th, and thought I could at least check it out. I was one of the first people there. No one was there, the cat van had a dead battery and no dogs had shown up yet. The phone rang and it said, "NEUROSURGERY OF SOUTH KANSAS"; I was shocked because it was a Saturday. I actually screenshotted this phone call afterward because of how unusual it was. I answered, and it was a lady from the clinic saying they were so busy she was working on a Saturday to get caught up and would

I be available for the two-part surgery on February 3rd and 10th? I had no idea how I was going to make it work with work but I said, "Yes !" I called my mom and we cried, I was in absolute disbelief.

After we hung up, I thought I would check out the adoption event one more time. I drove around and saw no dogs, but decided to park anyway. As I started walking towards the adoption tent, I saw a tail going a million miles a minute. I thought, "Who is attached to that tail?" I followed it and found a cute little beagle dachshund mix and that was that.

I took him home and we have been together since. My sister had told me she would help me with a dog if I found one, and she also fell in love with the little guy I named Cooper. She watched him while I was in Kansas, providing me with plenty of photos and videos.

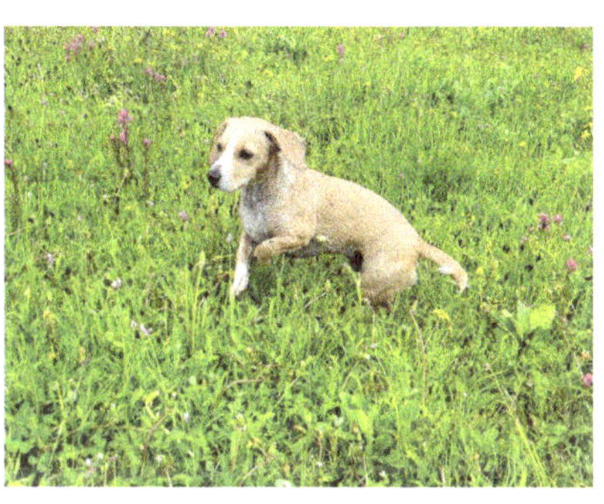

Cooper running through a field of wildflowers

38

Bri's Perspective

In the months leading up to surgery, knowing I would have to completely shave my head, I decided to go crazy with my hair trying things I never would have before. I had an amazing hair stylist who had been with me for a good decade of my journey, who helped me with these fun ideas. First, full blue, then a side shave, then both sides, the last was a buzz cut before the nurse took the last of my hair leaving me with a beautiful bald head. I am so glad she asked if I wanted a picture because it will never be that smooth again! Ha!

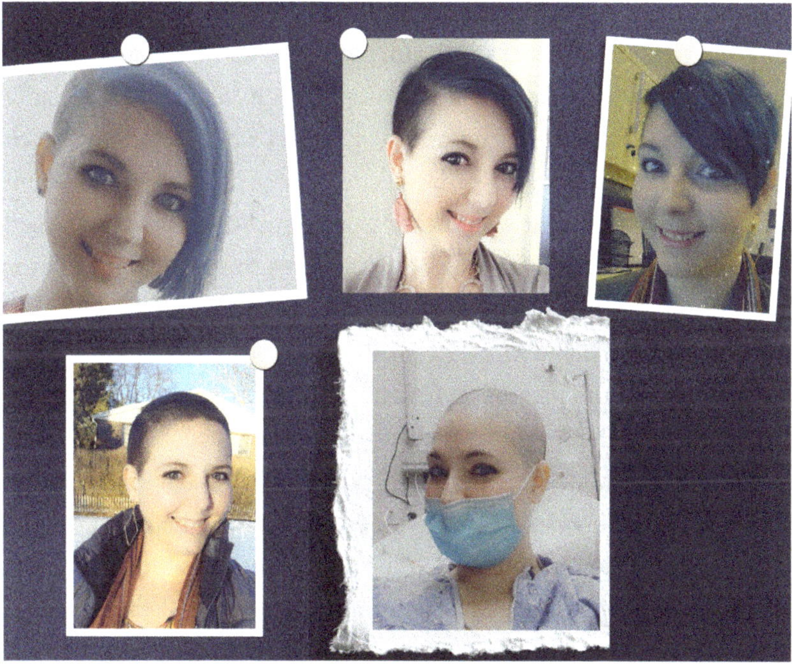

My hair transformation leading up to surgery

A Mama's Perspective

We took Bri to the hospital, Menorah in Overland Park, Kansas and dropped her off for her surgery. We were told that they would update us on their progress using text. Hours went by, 11 hours according to my timing. I thought that she had been in surgery for most of the 11 hours but this wasn't so. A lot of time had been just waiting for preparation. I later learned that her surgeon, Dr. C, performs surgeries from 6 am until midnight, or later, and is back again the next day. This little nugget of information was quite unsettling. You are working on my daughter's brain without much sleep and I am supposed to be excited about this? Around 4 pm we received a text that everything was going so well that they had asked Bri if she wanted to go ahead and have the battery stimulator implanted as well. She agreed. She had been awake for the lead placements and was doing extremely well so they all agreed to put her under general anesthesia for the battery implant. She received the Medtronic Percept non-rechargeable unit because, at this time, it had the most programming features. Around 7 pm we were allowed to see her. Her dad visited her the next day before his flight back home. Then I came to see her. She was a vision of ethereal beauty, her head bandaged in white gauze and her beautiful blue eyes just beaming. I had expected a bruised and very frail, tired, and uncomfortable daughter, instead, she was lovely and glowing.

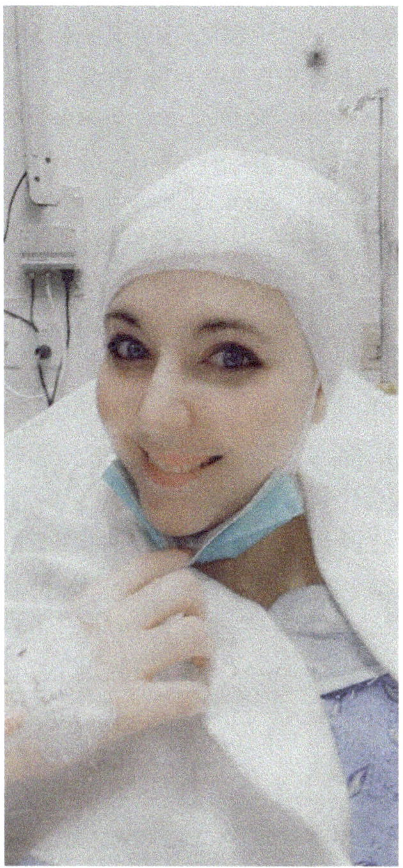

Smiling after waking up from brain
surgery

"A woman's strength isn't just about how much she can handle before she breaks, it's also about how much she must handle after she is broken."-Unknown

They had turned on her battery and she was experiencing what they call the "honeymoon phase" due to the brain swelling from surgery, where the symptoms of her disorder are basically non-existent, even before being programmed. They say this honeymoon phase can last up to three weeks. She stayed for three days before being released to go back to the rental home. I couldn't believe how well she was doing. On day five, she contacted work and started working remotely from Kansas City. Bri had her first programming a week after her surgery and it went really well. My brother had sent her a text with the meme of the New York Mets mascot, the baseball head with the red stitching, and he said, "The Mets want their mascot back." It was so funny because Bri's head was full of sutures and kind of reminded me of a baseball with its red stitches. We showed Dr. BAs my brother's text with pictures and he died laughing. He has an absolutely great sense of humor. Bri was feeling really well. We were taking walks around the neighborhood and walking to the various restaurants close by. She wasn't supposed to wear anything on her head, or cover her sutures with bandages, so she showed up in the restaurants in all of her glory. Several people inquired about her surgery. Around eight days after her surgery she was having difficulty with headaches and some bruising and swelling to one side of her temples. We called Meg and she said to go to the ER at Menorah, that they would know how to deal with Bri. She was kind enough to come and take Bri to the ER. Bri was given some medications for headaches and came home.

Bri then had another successful programming two weeks after her surgery. I asked Dr. BA different questions. He showed us various videos of the many kids he treats who have had DBS surgery and he has permission to share their journeys with others. A nine-year-old girl's video was very interesting. With her programming, she became so ecstatic and happy over everything. She was definitely on cloud nine; in love with everyone and everything. Dr. BA explained that this was actually a problem. I was perplexed because it sure didn't seem like a problem to me. He said it was a programming issue. Then he showed us several minutes later after she had had her settings changed. She had turned into a raging monster cursing at him and threatening him. I was so taken aback. He said that this was also a programming issue and that we should be very aware of emotional changes, that they might be due to needing a change in settings. These videos were very informative. Meg had shown me several of her videos before and after surgery. What a difference the surgery had made for her.

By week three, and Bri's last programming for a while, she was instructed on the parameters of her device and the range of settings she was given to use. She was allowed to go to 1.7v on the right side lead which controls her left side of her body and she was also allowed to go to 2.1v on the left side lead that controls the right side of her body. Bri also maintains a frequency between 130-160 hz. The unit was programmed so that she couldn't go any higher and Dr. BA joked, "You seem responsible."

I asked about the alcohol and Myoclonus Dystonia connection. Dr. BA pulled up some information on how the brain functions with Myoclonus Dystonia. We had also mentioned that Bri had never slept well, even with medication. Dr. BA showed us an image of a brain with Myoclonus Dystonia, its glucose consumption depicted in red; the entire brain was red. Then he showed us a normal brain and its consumption of glucose; there were just little pinpricks of red color here and there showing its glucose consumption. What a difference in the two images. My heart was heavy. I wondered if the Myoclonus brain craves alcohol because of the glucose consumption it requires, and if it is just a ravenous and insatiable monster for glucose, but the doctor wasn't sure about this theory. Dr. BA also explained to us how the brain in Myoclonus Dystonia is always in excitement mode and that it may mimic mania because it is just always being stimulated and is extremely excitable. This was heart-breaking to learn as well because a lot of Bri's drinking comes about because she's had very little, to no sleep and she just wants "lights out" for a day or two. By drinking in excess and passing out, she gets her wish, but when the alcohol wears off it sets off the anxiety aspect of the disorder along with the various physical rebound symptoms of the disorder. Then her brain is in wired and excitable mode again and wanting "lights out" again down the road. It is a vicious circle.

Bri's Perspective

I thought the nerves would hit me going into an awake brain surgery but instead, I just got happier and happier. There were still covid restrictions in place and my mom had a new puppy she brought with her so my parents dropped me off to get ready for surgery. It came time to shave my head and start an IV. The staff was fantastic and we were all joking around while they drilled little fiducials, or little titanium screws, into my skull to hold my head in place in a stabilizing halo for the surgery.

While the procedure is done awake, they gave me enough medication that I was not aware of the surgeon making the two holes through my skull. They then reduced the medication so I could interact with my neurologist to confirm they got the right placement of the two leads in the GPi (Globus Pallidus Internus-sounds like a Harry Potter spell!) part of my brain. Let me tell you, that was weird! While I had heard that the

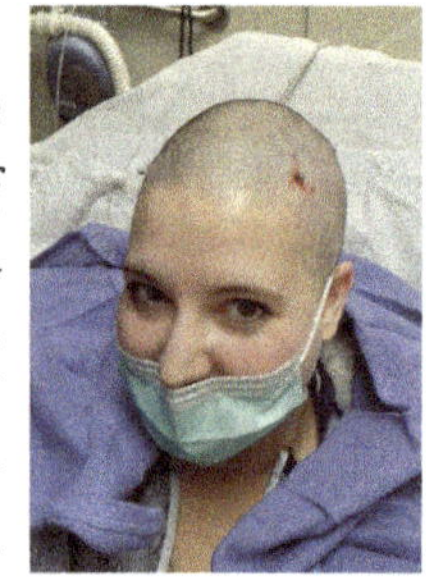

Placed fiduciaries for the stabilizing halo

brain does not have pain receptors, I was unaware you could actually feel what was going on in there. I still remember my surgeon adjusting my right lead. It was such a weird sensation having them dig around in my brain!

There were really only two bad parts to my surgery, the first bad part, was trying to communicate with a severely dry mouth. All the medications they were giving me left me with less moisture than a sun-bleached stone in the Sahara. I swear there was a nurse on standby just to feed me ice chips. The second uncomfortable part was by the end of the lead placements, my neck began to really hurt. Even when my doctor asked the anesthesiologist for something to help, it was still incredibly painful. I was so relieved when they asked if I was up for placing the battery right then too because I knew they'd knock me out for that part! After the neurostimulator battery was placed in my chest, the wires from the two leads were snaked through my skin down the side of my head and neck to connect to the battery. I ended up with three incisions on my scalp in addition to the screws and one on my chest. The first part of the surgery was only about three hours long, I was awake in recovery before 7 pm.

The surgery was incredible! People tell me it's like I got a second chance at life, or that it gave me my life back, to which I correct them by stating, "It gave me a life!" I'd been struggling for 20 years and I could finally go at life like an able-bodied person. Letting nothing slow me down, I returned to work full-time five days after surgery; I was back in the office in less than a month. I continued to push and excel at work despite a few setbacks from the surgery. I have always pushed and pushed and pushed. Just months after surgery, I started paddle boarding, I completed a 5k obstacle course, "The Muddy Dash," and I rode my bike again for the first time since Atlanta.

39

A Mama's Perspective

Bri was released to return home to Colorado and we had a 10-hour drive ahead of us. It had been snowing on and off in Kansas City during our stay. We headed out with about 2 feet of snow on the ground. I didn't know how Bri would travel but she did really well. We stayed the night in a hotel halfway back to Colorado, headed out the next day, making good time. We got Bri settled back into her apartment. She started going in to work only a short 21 days after having her surgery. Things went really well for the next three weeks; then she started having horrific headaches and had to go to the ER several times. They prescribed the headache medication, Butalbital, and she just suffered through daily headaches and still went to work.

Along with the headaches, about a month after surgery, she noticed one of her sutures was getting really red and irritated. Infection is a common complication of DBS surgery; it can comprise the whole unit making it necessary to remove everything. It can then be several months to over a year to heal before a second attempt. However, some people are not eligible to have the second surgery. Bri's PCP prescribed an antibiotic and had swabbed the suture area for cultures. Five days later, the culture also showed a fungal infection, so he ordered an antifungal and called it into the pharmacy. I was getting really nervous knowing these infections had been brewing for a while already, so I called the pharmacy to make sure we could pick it up that day. They told me it would be ready by 7 pm and the pharmacy hours listed said they were open until 9 pm. I arrived at 7:05 pm to find the security gate had been pulled down but the pharmacist and tech were still there. I asked if I could pick up the prescription and he said, "No, we're closed." I said it was an emergency and that my daughter had just received brain surgery and could lose her $275,000 system that she waited to receive for over 15 years. He was nasty and said he would put the already filled prescriptions back on the shelf and call the other King Soopers in town. It was going to take him more time to do this than just letting me get them then. I started to cry. I was exhausted and terrified that Bri could potentially lose everything not knowing if the infections were inching closer to her brain!

I drove to the other pharmacy crying and when I got there, it only took them 10 minutes to fill the script and they even saved me $500 by switching to a generic brand. The pharmacist consoled me and I thanked her. Bri started on the antifungal and antibiotic for the next 30 days and avoided a catastrophic failure. I saw this same pharmacist a month later and she asked how we were doing. We were doing great.

Several weeks into Bri's new daily headaches and working again full time, we decided that she needed to have some time to heal and she asked if she could work remotely for a few months. Her boss granted her request and she came home to Montrose where I could monitor her progress better and make her back off if needed.

Bri is also a commercial drone pilot and as part of her job, she was required to video job sites for the owners about every two weeks. We had worked out a schedule where I would drive her back to the front range for a few days so that she could shoot the videos. She started living with me on March 1, 2022 and had permission to work remotely, except for the droning once a month, until August. By June though, Bri was getting very antsy and she also had a Sarcoma follow-up in Denver for early June. Instead of driving her back and forth, she convinced me she would be okay to live with her dad again so we allowed her to go back to the front range to work full-time.

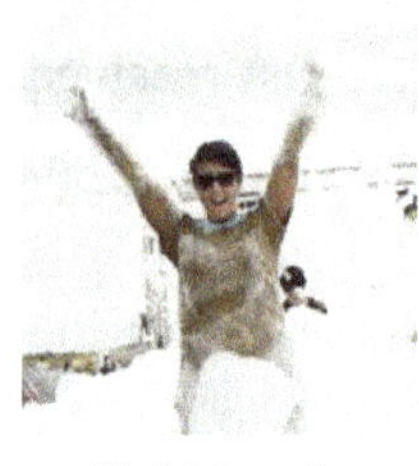

Finishing the Muddy Dash a few months after brain surgery

In June, she signed up for a 5K muddy obstacle course run with her sister and a friend. She completed the course with flying, muddy colors. Then she decided to buy herself a paddleboard and convinced her sister to buy one as well. They spent the summer paddle boarding on their days off. I couldn't believe the difference in Bri. In a few short months, she went from having tremors non-stop, difficulty walking, and an inability to negotiate stairs, to running obstacle courses and stand-up paddleboarding. Her mood had also improved and we were noticing that with her sleep medication, she was now getting almost eight hours of sleep frequently.

40

A Mama's Perspective

We were learning new things about life with DBS. Her settings had been stable for a few months, requiring very little change. However, one day, she said that she really wasn't feeling too well and that she was starting to twitch a bit. I asked her how much water she had drunk that day, as she generally drinks over 70 oz a day. She realized that she hadn't drunk any water, she'd been too busy; it was 5 pm. I said that I thought with the brain needing to be hydrated, and with the electrical impulses from the leads, that by being dehydrated it maybe created a "settings change". I suggested that she try drinking some water before trying to change her settings. She downed a few glasses of water; a few hours later she was feeling better. We realized over time that if she is ill with a fever that it will also cause what seems like a settings change. So she doesn't change her settings when she is ill, preferring to ride out her illness and then see how things are. We've also been fascinated to learn that Bri can now tolerate cold temperatures, they no longer set off twitching, tremors, or jerking anymore. She does notice a very weird feeling of "tightening", like her body would like to start having symptoms but it never gets to that point. We did notice that one day, she went without eating because her dad wanted to show a friend around the area and he didn't stop for food. Bri hadn't eaten since breakfast; as the day progressed, she started feeling ill. By 6 pm she was really twitching and I was horrified. Lesson learned, she needs to eat or her settings won't alleviate her symptoms.

41

A Mama's Perspective

Bri's dad was getting ready to retire (again) in the summer of 2022. He felt that the new owners of the company would more than likely let Bri go (cleaning house so to speak,) so he advised her that she might want to start looking for another position. As things would have it, she was immediately recruited for a position with a very large, and very old, national construction company as their marketing director and proposal writer. She would be working for a recent startup at an office in Castle Rock, Colorado. They made her a deal that she couldn't refuse. The pay was outstanding and the benefits were amazing. She would be at the top of the corporate ladder in her profession.

She was supposed to start her job on November 1, 2022. Bri had gone down to Castle Rock, met her boss in person, and then she'd gone to look at apartments. She chose an apartment that was only a half mile from the office so that she could start walking to work again. To say she was on cloud nine was an understatement. However, things would take a dramatic turn as she waited to start her new job.

I noticed that she still fatigued easily. She was still dealing with daily headaches. She had been prescribed Butalbital and was taking it daily to relieve her headaches although it didn't work all that well.

I hadn't realized that she had been getting more anxious about her job at her dad's company. Her immediate boss was difficult to work with and Bri just wasn't comfortable working for her boss the last few months before she accepted the new job. I didn't know that Bri's anxiety was really starting to ramp up.

She had given her three-week notice per her dad's request, but after the first week, her boss let her go. She had already packed to move; she was just waiting to start her new job. As the time slowly ticked by, she ended up getting really anxious. She didn't sleep for three nights in a row, trouble was brewing. Her dad had told her that if she lived with him, which she did, and if he caught her drinking, he'd throw her out. This was always heartbreaking to me because I viewed her drinking as part of her disorder. She was doing the best that she could at the time. However, I felt for my husband because she could really trash a place when she was intoxicated. He worked long hours and didn't need to come home to a disaster and a very drunk, if not passed out, daughter. It was truly heartbreaking seeing her in that condition. She'd come this far but there were still kinks to work out, why would we throw in the towel now? We had been told by her DBS neuro that he would never judge her for losing her sobriety, that it happens. I didn't want to enable her, but I also didn't want my beautiful daughter on the streets dealing with her rare disorder. Especially now, with a Deep Brain neurostimulator in her head and chest. She has never wanted to cause us any trouble. She truly has a beautiful disposition, has always been such a hard worker; she just needed more time to work things out.

She abruptly called me on a Wednesday night and said that she was going to go on a vacation for a few days to see more of Colorado. I thought this was very odd, she had packed up her dog and headed out at 7 pm that night for a mountain town about an hour away. She sent me pictures the next morning of her beautiful little bed and breakfast along the river so I thought maybe she really did need to get away before starting an intense new job. The next morning more pictures and she said she was going to stay another night. When she got back to the Greeley area, instead of going home where her dad was, she ended up in a hotel; I knew something was amiss. I called her and she confessed that she had been drinking. I packed my bags, packed up my puppy and we headed for the hotel. I had Tara stay with Bri until I could get to the hotel. I arrived about eight hours later; Bri was in bad shape. Bri and I had a long talk when I got there. I knew she was going to have a rough couple of days coming up and she was to start her new job just days after she would have detoxed. Not a great way to start a new job and the pressure she was facing wasn't going to help her heal. I was very adamant that she should think seriously about declining the new job and come home with me for at least a year to heal.

She hadn't taken much time to actually heal from her DBS surgery as she was back working remotely, and full-time, by day five and she was back in the office on day 21 after her surgery. Most people took up to six weeks off or they were on disability before their surgeries. I implored her to really think about taking on this new job with the hours and the stress involved, when she was still dealing with anxiety, sleep issues, frequent headaches, not to mention her unrelenting fatigue. I had learned that headaches and ongoing fatigue were something that people with DBS continue to deal with long after their surgeries.

Bri still wasn't sleeping and she cried for a week solid about the loss of her future; after having reached the pinnacle of her career. She was so excited to live on her own again and really make a name for herself in her career. Instead, with her in reluctant agreement, I had her call her new boss and decline the position due to health reasons. I tried to assure her that maybe the Universe had other plans for her and that with her brain always in excitement mode, that maybe a high-powered and stressful career wasn't the best choice to quiet an already overstimulated brain. It hadn't even been a year since her surgery and a lot of people I had met on the support groups for DBS were still struggling. I suggested that maybe Bri should turn to writing her stories as a cathartic outlet for what she was feeling. She had saved up a nice little nest egg and living with me, she wouldn't have too many expenses. She begrudgingly agreed to come home with me. Before I came back over to help her move, she'd already written her first book describing what had led to a near-death experience in 2017. I couldn't believe that she had written it in less than a week. Her brain definitely needed to be engaged with setting and reaching her goals.

42

Bri's Perspective

When it came time to move on from the company again, I was recruited to a "start-up" company with a huge, financially stable background. I had done it. I made it to the top of my career by age 31. I did it with Myoclonus Dystonia and brain surgery. I couldn't be more excited.

However, I was still extremely fatigued and while knowing I could do the job mentally, I wasn't sure if I could handle the stress of the first month of commuting a minimum of five hours through the Colorado winter season and through Denver and back home. On top of the drive, I would have a long workday for 45 days before I could move into my apartment.

I was allowed to leave a week early from my 3-week notice so I desperately wanted a vacation. I stayed a night in Denver, and two in Idaho Springs. When I got back, I had decided to drink because my anxiety was building and the hydroxyzine I took for anxiety wasn't cutting it. I went to stay the night at a hotel in Greeley. I came clean with my mom who then came and spoke with me that maybe it was finally time for me to find my calling. Every time I moved up on the corporate world path, the universe knocked me down. Cancer, Covid, Myoclonus Dystonia, etc. It was less than a year after a huge brain surgery so why didn't I give my body some time to heal? I figured it's now or never. I was raised to push through fatigue and work hard and climb the corporate ladder. I made it to the top, I had a huge surgery, and I am so much further along than many others suffering from this condition. I was offered a year at home to finish healing and maybe try something new. If I didn't find a new calling, I could go back to corporate America. Well, because my brain is set up to go-go-go, I have always given everything I've done intense effort and attention. I ended up writing the first draft of my first book in less than a week. I finished packing and moved to Montrose.

43

A Mama's Perspective

We got Bri moved over to Montrose and the next few weeks were full with her finishing her first book, editing it, and getting it published. "*White Flame*" is the title of her first book regarding her near-death experience in 2017.

On Oct 29, 2022, Bri and Tara flew out to see Dr. BA for a follow-up appointment and to get a wider range of settings available to her. With her initial visit, Dr. BA had her take the Cerebral Palsy genetic panel test because he could perform it for free, and he thought it might give him some information as to what gene/s might be involved in Bri's disorder.

Dr. BA is amazed by her response to the DBS surgery because he had only given her about a 60-75% chance of DBS alleviating her dystonia symptoms and he didn't have even that much hope for the myoclonic symptoms. It seems that the programming, with previous equipment, can either alleviate the dystonia, or the myoclonus, but not both at once with the same settings. However, he has been pleasantly surprised by Bri's response to the programming capabilities. She programs easily and it stays in a stable range of settings, offering her almost 98% improvement with her physical symptoms immediately, and over time with her psychological ones as well. With her Medtronic Percept neurostimulator, the electrical pulses can be directed in one direction or in a bubble-like fashion. One setting sent the pulse too close to the "capsule" and Bri immediately started to have twitching and dystonic sensations in her tongue, mouth, lips and face. It was a settings issue. Another setting had her on the verge of tears which is very unlike her. Again, it was a settings issue. It is fascinating how quickly changes can be felt with a settings change.

Dr. BA was very kind in answering some of our questions. I had stumbled upon the inhibitory response system, the proactive and reactive inhibitors. I was wondering how they might work in Myoclonus Dystonia. Dr. BA said that this was something that he was fascinated with and he was excited to explain things to Bri and her sister Tara. This is our rudimentary understanding of what he shared. The inhibitory processes, both the proactive and reactive processes are compromised in Myoclonus Dystonia. The limbic and caudate systems are designed to check on one another, keep a balance. It's as if one part of the inhibitory response is the character Tigger; over the top, very excitable, bouncy, going a million miles a minute, reckless, and impulsive. The other character is Eeyore; slow motion, no hurries, cautious. What the inhibitory process is supposed to do, is to bring Tigger and Eeyore more toward the middle, with Tigger slowing down and becoming more cautious and with Eeyore speeding up and being less cautious. They are supposed to balance each other out like a magnet that attracts each other to stick together in the middle. Instead, this process is failing in the Myoclonus Dystonia brain and the magnet poles are such that Tigger and Eeyore are being forcefully repelled away from each other and they are going further away from each other creating chaos. Tigger is getting crazier and Eeyore is becoming more and more lethargic.

With the Myoclonic brain, there is a measurable electrical excitability in the cortex, along with being very irritable. Usually the more irritable a brain is, the more it is prone to having seizure activity. However, in Myoclonus Dystonia, the individual doesn't have seizures and it's unknown why. The dopamine/GABAergic system isn't working correctly and it isn't tamping down the excitability of the cortex. It's the "perfect storm." DBS surgery stimulates the area where the excitability is coming from, interrupting its errant signals in an attempt to calm things down, telling Tigger to knock it off and Eeyore to get with the program.

Dr. BA also explained what is happening in the brain with the neurotransmitters and the axons. In a brain with Myoclonus Dystonia, the axons are shorter than a normal brain. When the neurotransmitter signals travel down the short axon, they have trouble reaching their intended target thus creating dystonic movements. Also, because the axon is too short, many of the neurotransmitters veer off course and end up affecting other areas that weren't expecting this neurotransmitter and this creates the Myoclonus because areas are getting excited messages. Dr. BA told her during this visit that a new gene had been located just three weeks earlier. He thinks in Bri's lifetime that there will be a possibility of a genetic therapy to cure her or others.

With the Cerebral Palsy panel, they found several genes from the paternal side that are mutated, so during this visit, he set Bri up with a geneticist and they are doing a more in-depth study. They are also testing her dad, her sister, and me. Hopefully, they may be on to finding a new gene for Myoclonus Dystonia.

We're excited to see how her brain will continue to respond to the electrical stimulation of the DBS unit and its building of new neurological pathways and lengthening the axons. We continue to be amazed at the activities that Bri now enjoys after having given up on them. We went on a recent hike, where just months prior to her DBS surgery, her vertigo and spastic movements had made it extremely difficult to walk down a set of steps along a hillside towards a river below. She clung to the hillside with me holding her arm on the other side and blocking her from falling. She was absolutely panicking during this hike. We revisited this hike after her DBS surgery and she not only went down the hillside towards the river without flinching, but she sassily walked back up the hill and walked up backwards!

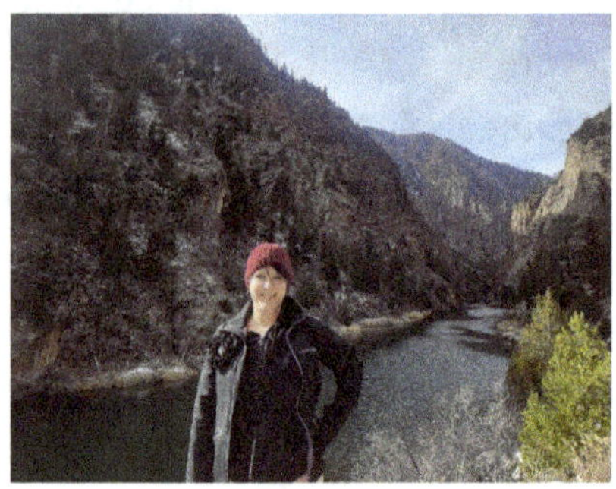

Repeating a hike at Black Canyon with success after DBS

Bri's Perspective

I love spending time with Dr. BA as he is full of information he enjoys sharing. During my fall follow-up, my sister joined me. I thought she would get a lot out of the visit because of her fascination with the brain. She is so fascinated with it that she got her master's degree in psychology. Tara summed up what he said, that her brain, "Is literally wired for dysfunction", hence the title of this book. After listening to my doctor's explanation of what was physically going on in the brain, I also came up with my own analogy for it. A car is driving down a road trying to get from point A to point B, but halfway down the road, it comes across a road-closed sign. Not knowing what to do, the car gets stuck and shakes as it idles trying to figure out the next move causing the dystonic symptoms. Meanwhile, the Myoclonus shouts "screw it!" and with its extra excitability, hits the gas and floors it through the road-closed sign. It ends up off of the road, not knowing where it's heading, bouncing around in a cornfield causing the myoclonic symptoms. The Deep Brain Stimulator comes and provides a detour for the car to get from point A to point B while constructing the rest of the road.

44

A Mama's Perspective

Looking back on our journey it's been bittersweet. I've witnessed a very beautiful and sweet soul, afflicted with a very difficult disorder that no one would wish on their worst enemy, try to navigate life to the best of her ability over the last 21 years. I have come to see her as a superhuman rockstar, unstoppable and with a heart full of wisdom and compassion. As a mom, it has been very challenging to witness the torment of a child so young and to realize that my lack of ability to comfort her was soul-crushing. In light of everything we've learned, I shouldn't be so harsh with myself. It is an extremely difficult disorder to deal with for both the sufferer and their loved ones.

I will also admit to being jealous of my friends with their children growing up with good friendships, great health, wonderful opportunities, and eventually marrying and having children of their own. Our lives have taken a very different path. There were so many nights that I was on my knees in prayer. Sometimes, I was very angry with God and I let Him know it. I am not ashamed of this because I know Him to be my Creator, and Father. He wants our honesty, so I let Him have it on more than one occasion. A few years before Bri's successful surgery, I had opened my bible randomly and found 2 Kings 20:5 "... I have seen thy prayer, I have seen thy tears: behold I will heal thee..." I was taught that every verse in the Bible is a promise and I claimed this promise for Bri. God did indeed hear my prayers eventually. She was given a life-saving surgery a few years later.

I also look back and see the strife between my husband and I, being at odds with one another on what steps to take next with a chronically ill child, without any good answers or effective treatments. I don't think my husband truly understood the gravity of Bri's disorder until the day she told him that she was approved for Deep Brain Stimulation surgery. It was also difficult knowing that Tara was suffering from MCAS-Mast Cell Activation Syndrome, POTS-Postural Orthostatic Tachycardia Syndrome and EDS-Ehlers Danlos Syndrome, the "Trifecta," and that she had been put on the back burner for so many years while I dealt with Bri's health issues.

During our journey, I would learn about the grief cycle, and how we are affected by our changing emotions on the roller coaster ride of chronic illness. The five emotions are: denial, anger, bargaining, depression, and acceptance. I would learn that rarely, if ever, any of us in our family would be feeling the same emotion at the same time. This made it difficult to understand one another until we looked at each other in a new light and the terms of the grief cycle. One day I might be in depression over the loss of Bri's future goal of being a world-class rock climber; my heart would be breaking for her. She would be in denial over the fact that she couldn't have a normal dinner out with a boyfriend. Then my husband might be feeling angry that as a family we were now dealing with alcohol abuse issues. Tara might be in acceptance mode that life was never going to be normal for her family. Any of us, and our emotions, could switch in a brief moment, changing the dynamics of our family and making it very difficult to navigate each emotional cycle with each other.

45

A Mama's Perspective

After Bri's successful surgery, I wrote an email to the DMRF to share briefly what a journey this has been. One of the board members received my email and she called to talk with me about how emotional she had gotten reading the letter. She ended up crying and had her husband read the email as well. Bri will hopefully be able to share more of her story in the future during a DMRF conference. We hope that she can speak specifically to the alcohol abuse feature of the disorder and how dangerous it is that some specialists still recommend drinking, "if it helps." I was just contacted by a mother of a 16-year-old girl with Myoclonus Dystonia that was just given this advice for her daughter by her specialist! This is unacceptable and we are trying to get the word out so that others won't suffer the same awful consequences that Bri has. The susceptibility to alcohol abuse with this disorder is said to be around 66%. The alcohol abuse feature of this disorder is why Dr. BAs prefers to intervene very early, before the preteens and teenagers find out what alcohol does to their symptoms (works extremely well at alleviating them) and also before their brain starts craving alcohol after having had it. It is still an occasional challenge for Bri, but she is doing much better with her sobriety.

Bri's Perspective

I think my family and I have gone through the grief cycles[17] hundreds of times; and I think we still do. I know I do. For what could have been, for what wasn't, for what did happen and so on. However, I am using this time my parents have been able to give me to get well in every aspect. Allowing my brain to heal from surgery and then allowing the DBS to create the neuro pathways needed to have a functional brain. Allowing my body to rest and recover from two decades of Myoclonus Dystonia battles. Allowing my spirit to tell me what my purpose is here on Earth. Right now, I am not focused on the past or too far into the future, so I can appreciate the now. One of my favorite sayings is, "If you have one foot in the future and one foot in the past, you're pissing on the present."

I also want to go into a life of helping others and that means that I have to help myself first. I am still working on the various techniques used to help in places that the DBS has not yet completely overcome. I want to get to a place where I can help others with these techniques. Of course, I also want to help others by getting information out there which is why my mom and I are co-authoring this book. We want to reach out to those affected by a rare disorder, whether it be a person suffering from it, or a caretaker advocating for their loved one, or a loved-one that is along for the difficult journey. This book is even for friends who just want to better understand so that they can be more supportive.

46

A Mama's Perspective

Bri continues to do well living in Montrose while pursuing a non-corporate, non-stressful lifestyle. Her brain is definitely starting to quiet down. We talked about taking the next year to "hack her brain" and see what techniques and/or therapies quiet her mind down. Maybe by always pushing so hard and working in stressful careers that are very stimulating, it is very difficult for her brain to quiet down. This exacerbates her anxiety and OCD levels which are features of her disorder. By living in the quiet little town of Montrose, away from any big city energy, she will eventually learn how to balance her mind. We hike daily and recharge in the peaceful quiet that surrounds us.

Since moving, she has discovered that Mindfulness Meditation has many different forms. The first form she was taught didn't work because she was supposed to mindfully observe her thoughts and let them go. We've since realized that this is not an easy task for a brain that is wired for excitability and OCD. By paying attention to those thoughts, it seemed to kick in her OCD and it was near impossible to let those thoughts go. The OCD feature of this disorder is probably also responsible for her lack of response to hypnotherapy. It is extremely difficult to quiet and focus a mind with Myoclonus Dystonia. We have found that a different type of Mindfulness

Meditation works for Bri, a more engaged and physical meditation like walking and hiking. We discovered a virtual reality (VR) headset and the TRIPP[18] app for meditative-like experiences. Anything, where she can concentrate 100% on one activity, is meditative for her. Bri also found the Beat Saber app for the headset and this really is helping her with managing her anxiety. The headset is working wonders for Bri, she really enjoys the interplay that seems to quiet her mind while she is actively engaged. It is a bit pricey upfront, but when you think about seeing a counselor once a week for the rest of your life, the cost is absolutely worth it. Plus, I'm having fun using it as well.

The best remedy of all has definitely been Bri's Deep Brain Stimulation surgery; it has worked much better than expected. The psychological features of the disorder still are a work in progress, but we have already seen a great improvement there. We also found our dream doctor in Dr. BA, he enjoys picking our brains and offering us interesting tidbits about what he is finding out about Myoclonus Dystonia. I think he likes visiting with Bri because she is an adult and can give him really good information as to how her neurostimulator is working, whereas the kids in his practice might have a difficult time communicating exactly what they are trying to tell him. Her neurostimulator has the ability to capture data and this data can be transferred to researchers. Her neurostimulator has the ability to record all brainwave activity. Dr. BA sends information from Bri's unit to researchers when she has her follow-up visits. After the release of this book, we should have more genetic testing information, so that is exciting. Finally, we have a partnership with a doctor that we can trust and he is so much fun to visit with because he shares a lot of information and has a great sense of humor.

47

A Mama's Perspective

I feel like I have come full circle, from naive, to frustrated and scared, to vindicated and powerful. I am a great advocate for my daughters. I have also put my skills to use in the various support groups that I belong to, sharing what I have learned without giving medical advice. I also support those who are really facing difficult challenges with the open door invitation to direct message me or even call me if they need to and at any time of day, or night, and I mean it. I know how lonely and scared we can be and I don't want anyone to suffer in silence.

I also tell people to get another opinion, and another if necessary, until they finally have their answers and relief. I suggest people join the various support groups that are available, that they have a wealth of information, and sometimes, if not most times, the people know more about their conditions than their doctors. They also seem to have a wealth of up-to-date information and links to research and articles on the various disorders and the treatments and medications that are effective. They are all very supportive.

I also remind people that if things change in the future, they might need to revisit things and get yet another opinion as medical technology and knowledge is rapidly changing all of the time. I also tell them to trust their gut instinct and to keep going until their "radar" is satisfied with the answers and to not accept a medical professional that gaslights them. Doctors actually work for us but some of them forget that they do. You are able to fire them and find one who will work with you and respect you!

I definitely look upon this journey as a bittersweet blessing. I've learned a tremendous amount about myself, referring to myself as a "wingman" for Bri and Tara.

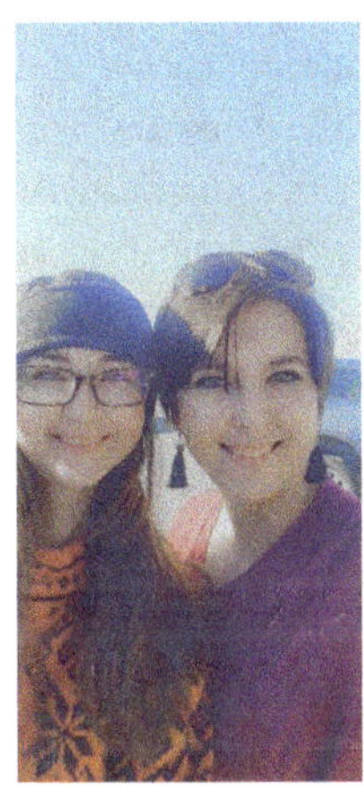

Bri and Tara, two Zebras

I've realized how special my strong, determined, tenacious, and indestructible Bri is. Tara is facing her own challenges with strength and resilience. I describe myself as a Zebra mom because that is what we call people with rare disorders. From the Arkansas Gazette, Little Rock, AR, (October 1962) "When you hear hoofbeats in the middle of the night, you look for horses, not zebras. In the rare disorder community, we affectionately refer to those who have rare disorders as zebras. The doctors are often looking for horses and it can take many years, to several decades to get a proper diagnosis because doctors aren't looking for "zebras."

I wish you the very best in your journeys. Stay strong and be your best advocate or have someone you trust to advocate for you.

Epilogue

The last two decades have been one heck of a wild ride and not always in a good way. I could not have made it to where I am now without my amazing mom and her refusal to give up, the forgiving nature of my sister, the financial and loving support of my dad, my angel Meg, and of course the neurological team I finally ended up with for my life altering DBS surgery. Writing this book has been extremely difficult for me as I have spent two decades hiding my symptoms, pushing forward as a "normal" person, and being in denial. Now that I have gotten some great help, I want to push past my own boundaries and share my story to help others out there. Writing this book alongside my mom has brought me so many tears as the feelings I repressed for decades came up. Sitting in corners of coffee shops with tears in my eyes, I finally was able to complete this story. Rereading this all at once made me realize why my sister says this is a story of resilience. My mom never gave up searching for answers and solutions, and even through the darkness, I see where I continued to fight and never truly gave up. Our story is still in its infancy as the DBS works to rewire my brain to be functional and life is revealing itself to me every day. I have been so blessed and I want to pass that blessing along, whether it's in the form of hope, understanding, or perhaps just some of the research we have come across in our journey and with my lived experiences.

"Every day I feel is a blessing from God. And I consider it a new beginning. Yeah, everything is beautiful."-Prince

Endnotes

1 Mayoclinic.org (May 4, 2022) Definition: "Essential tremor is a nervous system (neurological) disorder that causes involuntary and rhythmic shaking. It can affect almost any part of your body, but the trembling occurs most often in your hands-especially when you do simple tasks, such as drinking from a glass or tying a shoelace." I knew that Bri was also having muscle cramping and spasticity, so this diagnosis didn't quite fit either.

Mayoclinic.org (March 1, 2022) Definition: "Restless Leg Syndrome (RLS) is a condition that causes an uncontrollable urge to move the legs, usually because of an uncomfortable sensation. It typically happens in the evening or nighttime hours when you're sitting or lying down. Moving eases the unpleasant feeling temporarily." Although Bri had the sensation of body parts wanting to move, it wasn't the same as with RLS, so I discounted this diagnosis as well. It also didn't explain the other myriad of symptoms.

2 Mayoclinic.org (January 13, 2023)

3 Following the Equator: A Journey Around the World, 1897, Chapter 15

4 If you want to know more about this particular entity, Google: "Tall, evil, Shadowman with a top hat and a cape" or "phantom hat man" and you will find many resources describing this entity.

5 You can read all about the paranormal events and other frequencies experienced throughout Bri's life in her first book titled, "White Flame", in which she shares how she came to have a Near Death Experience (NDE) on April 27, 2017

6 EMcrit.org (May 1, 2022) "Catatonia is a motor dysregulation syndrome involving difficulty in initiating or terminating actions… Stupor."

7 Mayoclinic.org (January 11, 2022) Definition of Functional neurological disorder/conversion disorder: "A newer and broader term that includes what some people call conversion disorder-features nervous system (neurological) symptoms that can't be explained by a neurological disease or other medical

condition." However, the symptoms are real and cause significant distress or problems functioning.

8 Mayoclinic.org (January 11, 2022) Definition of Conversion Disorder: "Also known as functional neurological system disorder, it is a condition in which a person experiences physical and sensory problems, such as paralysis, numbness, blindness, deafness or seizures, with no underlying neurologic pathology."

9 According to AlcoholicAnonymous.com (February 24, 2022) 14 drinks per week is a level where females are considered an alcoholic.

10 According to information from the Dystonia Medical Research Foundation (DMRF) at dystonia-foundation.org, which we highly recommend, "Alcohol is a depressant, which means it slows the function of the central nervous system. Alcohol acts on the brain in ways that, over time, can degrade its ability to make muscles relax-which is already a problem for those with Myoclonus Dystonia. Long-term use of alcohol ultimately reduces the effects of alcohol and makes certain medications less effective. The combination of alcohol and medications can be damaging or deadly." This doesn't go into the other dangers of liver disease and liver failure/death, gastrointestinal damage, heart issues, brain damage, along with the other problems like the social, emotional, and financial damages. "The DMRF is a 501(c)(3) non-profit organization dedicated to advancing research for more dystonia treatments and ultimately a cure, promoting awareness, and supporting the well-being of affected individuals and families." You can find DMRF on Facebook, Twitter, and Youtube or https://www.dystonia-foundation.org

11 Epilepsy.com defines PME as "a group of more than 10 rare types of epilepsies that are "progressive." People with PME have a decline in motor skills, balance and cognitive function over time…they also have a shortened life span."

12 If you would like to know about the Near Death Experience and other phenomena, the International Association for Near Death Studies is a 501 (c)(3) non-profit organization for the research and study of near deaths along with education and support.

13 Mayoclinic.org (April 9, 2022) Definition:: "Ataxia describes poor muscle control that causes clumsy voluntary movements. It may cause difficulty with walking and balance, hand coordination, speech and swallowing, and eye movements."

14 If you'd like to take a peek at her wonderful food blog and what she ate, go to: https://brilafferty.wixsite.com/fantabulousfoods

15 For information on DBS go to Mayoclinic.org>test-procedures>deep-brain-stimulation>about>pac-20384562 and Medtronic.com

16 the principal inhibitory neurotransmitter in the Central Nervous System-https://doi.org/10.1073/pnas.0915139107

17 the Kubler-Ross Grief Cycle (https://grief.com)

18 the Meta 2 Oculus (https://www.meta.com/products); (https://tripp.com)

Contact Information

You can find links to many of the resources that have helped us on our journey on my website, www.Bri0nicLLC.com. I try to keep it updated with resources, youtube videos, DBS information, alcoholism, and much more.

You may reach out to Jill Lafferty at email: heavenlyhavens@msn.com or find her on Facebook to Private Message her.

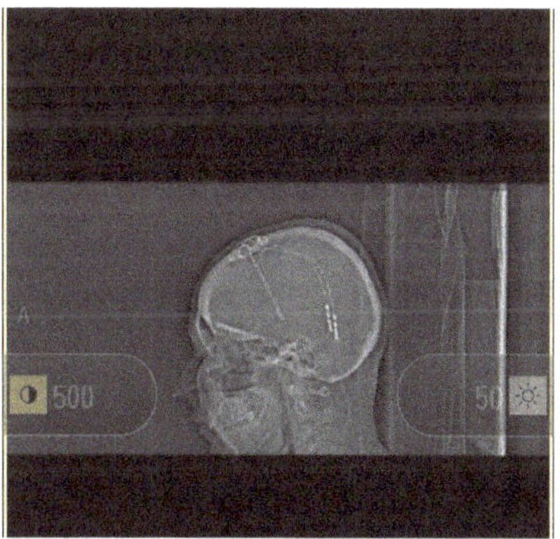

"I have innies, not outies", our joke about Bri being an alien with antennas. This is my CT scan to prove it.

Resources

RESOURCES

Alcoholics Anonymous   https://www.aa.org

Bri0nicLLC.com Bri's website (Bri0nic is with a zero)

Centers for Disease Control (CDC)   https://www.cdc.gov

Chris Hill (for Addictions)   https://seven-day-beat-addiction-plan.teachable.com

Depression https://www.nimh.nih.gov/health/topics/depression

Dystonia Medical Research Foundation (DMRF) a 501c (3) non-profit organization dedicated to serving families with dystonia.

https://www.dystonia-foundtion.org

1 E Wacker Drive, Suite 1730, Chicago, IL 60601 phone: (312) 755-0198

Please visit DMRF's website for more information on the various dystonias, their symptoms, diagnosis, treatments, how they affect your life, and current research and events.

Embraced by the Light. Betty Jean Eddie. Onjinjinkta Publishing, December 1992.

EMcrit.org Definition of Catatonia May 1, 2022

Dying to be Me. Anita Moorjani. Hay House. March 2012

Following the Equator: A Journey Around the World. Mark Twain. Hartford: American Publishing, 1897

Get Your Life Back: The Road to Freedom from Addiction. Chris Hill. Create Space Independent Publishing Platform. September, 26, 2016.

heavenlyhavens@msn.com Jill Lafferty email. You can also find Jill on Facebook

https://brilafferty.wixsite.com/fantabulousfoods Bri's website for her food blog

International Association for Near Death Studies (IANDS)
https://www.iands.org
2741 Campus Walk Avenue, Building 500, Durham, NC 27705-8878 phone: 1-919-383-7940
This organization is a 501c (3) non-profit dedicated to research, education, support, and resources.
You can also find IANDS on Youtube and Facebook. There are many sharing groups on Facebook.

Kubler-Ross Grief Cycle https://grief.com

Lifering Secular Recovery (for Alcohol Addiction)   a 501c (3) non-profit
https://lifering.org
25125 Santa Clara Street, E-359, Hayward, CA 94544 phone: 1-800-811-4142
service@lifering.org

Malingering   https://www.ncbi.nlm.nih.gov/books/NBK507837

Mast Cell Activation Syndrome mastcellaction.org

Mayo Clinic https://www.mayoclinic.org
https://www.mayoclinic.org/diseases

Medical Dictionary for definitions. https://medical-dictionary.thefreedictionary.com

Medtronic https://www.medtronic.com
710 Medtronic Parkway, Minneapolis, MN 55432-5605 phone: 1-800-633-8766

Merriam-Webster Dictionary for definitions. https://www.merriam-webster.com

Miracles from Heaven. Christy Wilson Beam. Hachette Books; Reprint Edition. November 17, 2015.

Myoclonus Dystonia Additional Resources:
https://medlineplus.gov/genetics/condition/myoclonus-dystonia
https://orpha.net
https://rarediseases.info.nih.gov

National Organization for Rare Disorders (NORD)
https://www.rarediseases.org
1900 Crown Colony Drive, Suite 310, Quincy, MA 02169 phone: (617)-249-7300

Ncbi.nlm.nih.gov National Center for Biotechnology Information, the National Library of Medicine, and the National Institute of Health.
NLM The National Library of Medicine, 8600 Rockville Pike, Bethesda. MD 20894
NIH The National Institute of Health, 9000 Rockville Pike, Bethesda, MD 20892 phone: (301)-496-4000

Never Bet Against Occam. Dr. Lawrence Afrin. Sisters Media, LLC, 1st Edition. March 15, 2016.

Occam's Razor https://conceptually.org>

Oxford English Dictionary for definitions. https://www.oed.com

Panic Attacks https://careinfo.mayoclinic.org/mental-health-anxiety

Post Traumatic Syndrome https://careinfo.mayoclinic.org

POTS-Postural Orthostatic Tachycardia Syndrome https://mycleveland-clinic.org/health/diseases/16560-postural-orthostatic-tachycardia-syndrome-pots

Pubmed.gov More than 35 million citations for biomedical literature from MEDLINE, life science journals, and online books. Part of the National Library of Medicine (NLM)

Sarcoma Alliance (Soft Tissue Sarcoma)
https://sarcomaalliance.org
775 E. Blithedale Avenue, #334, Mill Valley, CA 94941 phone: (415)-381-7234
info@sarcomaalliance.org

Sinclair Method (for Alcohol Cessation)
https://www.sinclairmethod.org
1455 NW Leary Way #458, Seattle, WA 98107 phone: 1-888-323-0575
Email: info@sinclairmethod.org

SMART Recovery (for Alcohol Addiction)
https://smartrecovery.org
7304 Mentor Avenue, Suite F, Mentor, OH 44060 phone: (440)-951-5357

Traumatic Brain Injury (TBI) https://www.alz.org

White Flame. 1048 BL, Brianna Lafferty. Bri0nic LLC, November 11, 2022.

Zebra Story. *When You Hear Hoofbeats.* Arkansas Gazette, Little Rock, AR. October 1962

One of the most beneficial therapies that I have found for remaining sober is Chris Hill's talking or writing a letter to your subconscious, communicating with it on a frequent basis to get its cooperation in helping you remain sober. You can find his information at: https://seven-day-beat-addiction-plan.teachable.com Along with Chris Hill's techniques, Dr. BAs supports Biofeedback and EMDR therapies because they help us sense when our brains are starting to ramp up and get too excitable. EMDR forces the brain to deal with its traumas when it wants to shut down instead. Otherwise, the brain just goes and goes while ignoring trauma until it crashes. It's like the myoclonus brain gets signals that the "bridge is out" up ahead but unless we have techniques to deal with this warning, we end up going over the edge and crashing.

List of Medication Bri Tried

MEDICATIONS LIST

Included in this medication list are the various medications that Bri was prescribed over the years. Before and after being properly diagnosed with Myoclonus Dystonia, she was put on medication "cocktails," sometimes as many as seven different prescriptions at a time and all at once instead of adding one and then another. This made it extremely difficult to monitor for side effects. With Myoclonus Dystonia, Bri had very little relief with the various combinations of medications and this is why she was a great candidate for Deep Brain Stimulation surgery, the medications failed to bring relief of her many symptoms.

We have only listed the side effects that were more common and experienced by Bri and the side effects that made it a challenge in deciphering whether it was a medication causing a symptom or exacerbating an already present symptom such as muscle rigidity, tremors, seizures, headaches, etc.

We used RxList.com to compile the information on the various medications that Bri was prescribed. Please note that there is a lot more information on RxList.com for the specific medications, their actions, their side effects and serious warnings if you would like more information about a certain medication.

Brand names may differ depending on the manufacturers.

The medications are listed in alphabetical order according to their generic names and they are not listed in a timeline sequential order of when Bri was prescribed a medication.

Again, this list of medications is for informational purposes only and is not to be taken as medical advice. Seek professional medical care for any medication needs.

It is a very good idea to keep a good notebook on medications. Log the name of the medications (both generic and brand name), what the medication is for, the dosage and how to take it, how many times a day to take the medication, when you started the medication, and any side effects that you may be experiencing along with your pharmacy contact information. Do not be afraid to tell the doctor that you think a medication is giving you a side effect or interacting with another medication that you are on. Also, sometimes a brand name will work better over the generic. Sometimes a manufacturer difference will make a difference as well or just a change in ingredients. For example, Bri didn't respond well to Relpax, Frova, or Maxalt (all "triptans") and yet Sumatriptan works very well for her, so a medication change just might make a difference overall.

Generic Name: Alcohol / Ethanol

Brand Name: Alcohol

Drug Class: Central Nervous System Depressant

Used For: Relief of myoclonus dystonia symptoms, especially the myoclonic jerking

Common Side Effects: feelings of relaxation or drowsiness, a sense of euphoria or giddiness, changes in mood, lowered inhibitions, impulsive behavior, slowed or slurred speech, nausea and vomiting, diarrhea, head pain, changes in hearing, vision, and perception, loss of coordination, trouble focusing or making decisions, loss of consciousness or gaps in memory (often called a blackout)

Serious Side Effects: Long-term use can lead to pancreatitis, alcohol-related liver disease, permanent brain damage, Ulcers, Circulatory system complications, bone density issues, anxiety, Dependence, withdrawal

*After reading through this list of medications, keep in mind, Bri didn't expect to live a long life so the short-term side effects of alcohol made sense as she couldn't foresee living long enough to experience the long-term side effects.

Generic Name: Alprazolam

Brand Name: Xanax

Drug Class: Benzodiazepine, Anxiolytic, Antianxiety

Used For: Anxiety, Sedative

Common Side Effects: Pounding heartbeat, drowsiness, slurred speech, convulsions/seizures

Serious Side Effects: Depressed mood, suicidal thoughts, tremor, uncontrolled muscle movements

(As you can see, there are several side effects that would look like symptoms of Myoclonus Dystonia and you will find this throughout this medications list)

Generic Name: Amitriptyline
Brand Name: Elavil
Drug Class: Tricyclics
Used For: Anxiety, depression, Bipolar, Depression
Side Effects: Shaking, muscle spasms, seizures, muscle stiffness, irregular heartbeat

Generic Name: Baclofen
Name Brand: Baclofen
Drug Class: Skeletal Muscle Relaxant
Used For: Muscle rigidity, muscle spasms, pain, clonus
Side Effects: tired, drowsiness, insomnia, nausea

Generic Name: Bupropion
Name Brand: Wellbutrin
Drug Class: Atypical Antidepressant, Dopamine Reuptake Inhibitor
Used For: Major Depressive Disorder, Seasonal Affective Disorder
Side Effects: Increased seizures/convulsions, mood/behavior changes, fast/irregular heartbeat, severe sleep problems, nausea, vomiting, tremors, anxiety/nervousness
Serious Side Effects: Warning Box: Suicidal thoughts and behaviors

Generic Name: Buspirone
Name Brand: Buspar
Drug Class: Antianxiety, non-benzodiazepine, anxiolytic
Used For: Anxiety
Side Effects: Headaches, drowsiness, nausea, feeling nervous

Generic Name: Butabital
Brand Name: Fioricet
Drug Class: Barbituate, narcotic, anxiolytic-hypnotic-anticonvulsant
Used For: Relieves tension headaches

Side Effects: A very long list. Addiction potential, life threatening overdose potential

***Bri uses this medication occasionally when she gets a really bad headache and it seems to work well for her without any side effects.

Generic Name: Carbamazepine
Brand Name: Tegretol
Drug Class: Antimanic Agent, anticonvulsant, Bipolar Disorder Agents
Used For: Epilepsy, neuralgia, Bipolar mania
Side Effects: Rapid heartbeat, unusual tiredness, headache, confusion, severe weakness, increased seizures, problems with balance/walking/coordination
Warning Box: See RxList.com

Generic Name: Carbidopa/levodopa
Brand Name: Sinemet
Drug Class: Decarboxylase Inhibitor
Used For: To increase dopamine neurotransmitters, muscle stiffness, tremors, spasms, poor muscle control.
Side Effects: Uncontrolled muscle movements of the face, eyes, lips, worsening tremors, rigid muscles, muscle contractions, somnolence
Movement Disorder Specialists should give anyone with dystonia symptoms a trial of this medication because if it is a "dopa-responsive" dystonia, this medication works really well to alleviate symptoms.

Generic Name Clindamycin HCL
Brand Name: Cleocin Hydrochloride
Drug Class: Antibiotic, Lincosamide
Used For: Treats a wide variety of bacterial infections
Side Effects: Nausea, vomiting, hives, diarrhea, trouble breathing, yeast overgrowth

Generic Name: Clonazepam
Brand Name: Klonopin
Drug Class: Anxiolytic, Benzodiazepine, Anticonvulsant
Used For: Seizures, panic disorder
Side Effects: Increased seizures, severe drowsiness, pounding heartbeat, unusual involuntary eye movements, problems with balance and coordination.

***This medication is usually a first line medication used to treat Myoclonus Dystonia but it left Bri feeling like a complete zombie and really out of it, drowsy, uncoordinated, brain fog. She really hated being on this medication and it really didn't alleviate any of her symptoms.

Generic Name: Cyclobenzaprine
Brand Name: Flexeril
Drug Class: Skeletal Muscle Relaxant
Used For: Muscle spasms (not effective for muscle spasticity)
Side Effects: Fast irregular heartbeat, slurred speech, drowsiness, headaches, nausea, balance problems

***(Should not be used long term) Bri still uses this medication occasionally and without side effects

Generic Name: Diazepam
Brand Name: Valium
Drug Class: Benzodiazepine, anxiolytic, anticonvulsant, skeletal muscle relaxant
Used For: Seizures, anxiety, muscle spasms, alcohol withdrawal, sedation
Side Effects: Anxiety, panic attacks, trouble sleeping, hyperactivity, worsening seizures, severe drowsiness, and a long list of other side effects.
Warning Box: Suicidal Thoughts and Behaviors

Generic Name: Divalproex
Brand Name: Depakote
Drug Class: Anticonvulsant
Used For: Seizures
Side Effects: Anxiety, panic attacks, trouble sleeping, nausea, weight gain, tremors, headaches,
worsening seizures, depression and a long list.
Warning Box: Life threatening adverse reactions, see list on RxList.com

***Bri was gaining one pound a day for 30 days on this medication, so it was discontinued. However, it wasn't relieving any of her symptoms either.

Generic Name: Duloxetine
Brand Name: Cymbalta

Drug Class: Serotonin and Norepinephrine Reuptake Inhibitor (SNRI), Antidepressant

Used For: Major Depressive Disorder, neuropathic pain, general anxiety, fibromyalgia, muscle pain

Side Effects: Pounding heartbeat, headaches, confusion, slurred speech, severe weakness, loss of coordination, insomnia

Warning Box: Suicidal Thoughts and Behaviors. Bri quickly had suicidal thoughts while taking Cymbalta

This is a medication that while trying to discontinue, you should ask your doctor about titrating down.

Generic Name: Eletriptan hydrobromide
Brand Name: Relpax
Drug Class: Antimigraine, Serotonin-5-HT –Receptor Agonist
Used For: Migraines
Side Effects: Rapid weight gain, headaches, nausea, anaphylactic reactions.

Generic Name: Escitalopram Oxalate
Brand Name: Lexapro
Drug Class: Selective Serotonin Reuptake Inhibitor (SSRI), Antidepressant
Used For: Depression, Major Depressive Disorder, general anxiety
Side Effects: Headaches, slurred speech, weakness, vomiting, drowsiness, anxiety, insomnia, tremors, muscle rigidity

Generic Name: Fluconazole
Brand Name: Diflucan
Drug Class: Antifungal systemic
Used For: Fungal infections
Side Effects: Pounding heartbeat, body aches, seizures, nausea, diarrhea, tremor, stomach pain
Severe Warning: See RxList.com

Generic Name: Frovatriptan Succinate
Brand Name: Frova
Drug Class: Antimigrain Agents, Serotonin 5-HT-Receptor Agonist
Used For: Migraines
Side Effects: See RxList.com-long list of side effects

Generic Name: Gabapentin

Brand Name: Neurontin
Drug Class: GABA-Analog, antiepileptic
Used For: Nerve pain, seizures
Side Effects: Increased seizures, problems with balance, uncontrolled muscle movements and rapid eye movements, swelling, headaches, drowsiness, eye problems, nausea
Serious Side Effects: Suicidal Behaviors, Withdraw from medication can precipitate seizures

***This medication within 2 months of starting it, caused Bri to have absence seizures with loss of bladder control, hallucinations, sleep walking and black out seizures. Her first black out seizure occurred while she was driving and she totaled her car. She was sent to an Epileptic Monitoring Unit but she had discontinued this medication prior to her three day stay. With discontinuation of this medication, Bri didn't have any more side effects. We reported this serious side effect to the FDA's Medwatch program. If you ever encounter a side effect that you think is dangerous, you can report it to the FDA Medwatch program and hopefully, in the future, they will take action to remove a dangerous drug.

Generic Name: Hydrocodone/APAP
Brand Name: Vicodin
Drug Class: Analgesic, Opioid Combination
Used For: Pain
Side Effects: Nausea, drowsiness, headaches
Warning Box: Misuse, Abuse, Life Threatening, Depression, Addiction

Generic Name: Hydroxyzine
Brand Name: Vistaril
Drug Class: Antiemetic, Piperazine Derivative, 1st Generation Antihistamine
Used For: Anxiety, Itching
Side Effects: Tremor, drowsiness, pounding heart, headache, seizures

***Bri still takes this occasionally and without any side effects. Before DBS, it quickly reduced her myoclonus symptoms for a time.

Generic Name: Imipramine
Brand Name: Tofranil
Drug Class: Antidepressant, TCAs
Used For: Depression

Side Effects: Anxiety, panic attacks, insomnia, balance and speech issues, seizures, pounding heartbeat
Serious Side Effects: Suicidal Thoughts

Generic Name: Levetiracetam
Brand Name: Keppra
Drug Class: Ligands, Anticonvulsants
Used For: Partial onset seizures, tonic-clonic seizures, myoclonic seizures
Side Effects: Depression, anxiety, extreme drowsiness, loss of balance and coordination, somnolence
Warning Box: Behavioral Abnormalities, Psychotic Symptoms, Suicidal Ideation

***Within two weeks of starting this medication, Bri was suicidal and her doctor had her discontinue and the side effect of suicidal ideation ceased. Scary though. This is why I highl6y recommend keeping a medication journal, so that if a medication becomes dangerous, you know which one and can alert your medical providers of how you react to a particular medication.

Generic Name: Levothyroxine sodium
Brand Name: Synthroid
Drug Class: Thyroid Product
Used For: Hypothyroidism, goiter   ***Dr. RJ was using it off label for Bipolar Disorder
Side Effects: Tremors, irregular heartbeat, tiredness, insomnia, increased depression, headaches, Leg cramps, muscle aches

Generic Name: Lorazepam
Brand Name: Ativan
Drug Class: Benzodiazepine, anxiolytic, anticonvulsant, works on neuro-transmitter GABA-A
Used For: Anxiety, sedation, seizures
Side Effects: Increased sleep problems, drowsiness, muscle weakness, slurred speech, lack of balance and coordination, memory problems
Warning Box: Suicidal Ideation

Generic Name: Methotrexate
Brand Name: Trexall
Drug Class: Antineoplastics, Antimetabolite, DMARDs, Immunomodulators

Used For: Chemotherapeutic agent for cancer in combination with other cancer therapies

Side Effects: See RxList.com, serious side effects, a long list of side effects

Generic Name: Modafinil

Brand Name: Provigil

Drug Class: Stimulant, CYP3AF Inducers-Moderate

Used For: Treating excessive sleepiness, narcolepsy, and shift work sleep disorder

Side Effects: Depression, anxiety, suicidal thoughts and actions, nausea, dizziness, insomnia

Serious Side Effects: See list at RxList.com

Warning Box: Serious, see RxList.com

***Bri 's neuropsychiatrist put her on this medication. It made a huge difference in her alertness and she seemed to really do well on it. However, when she saw the movement disorder specialist/psychiatrist after her first rehab stay, and she asked about if she could have a refill, it may have been a factor in her abrupt discharge with this particular doctor. Just a word of caution, we have since learned that this particular drug, Provigil, may get you labeled with "drug seeking behavior". We had no idea, and yet this drug really gave Bri the alertness to work full time and go to school without any side effects. Notice how many medications Bri was prescribed over the years have side effects of drowsiness.

Generic Name: Montelukast sodium

Brand Name: Singulair

Drug Class: Leukotrine Receptor Antagonist

Used For: Asthma, rhinitis, exercised induced bronchospasms

Side Effects: Unusual change in mood, pain, muscle weakness, headaches

Warning Box: Suicidal Ideation Behaviors Actions

***After three months of being on Singulair, Bri quickly became depressed, severely, and in just a few short days was suicidal and she had acted on it landing her in a three day psych ward hold. Being in a psych ward was absolutely terrifying for Bri and there were no avenues to get her out early, she just had to suffer in the ward where frightening behaviors were exhibited. We had been warned about mood changes and to be aware of them. There was also a warning on the prescription bottle regarding Suicidal Ideation. However, Bri was living on her own and out of town, when things just progressed very quickly.

Please be aware of this particular medication, in my opinion, it is very dangerous and not worth taking. We made a report to the FDA Medwatch program for Singulair regarding the reaction Bri experienced even though it is a known and posted serious side effect. Reporting any serious event may eventually get this drug taken off of the market. I have heard many heartbreaking stories of parents losing their children, even young adult children, to this medication when everything seemed fine and then out of nowhere, they took their lives.

Generic Name: Naltrexone Hydrochloride
Brand Name: Naltrexone Hydrochloride
Drug Class: Opioid Antagonist
Used For: Treatment of Alcohol Dependence
Side Effects: See Precautions

Generic Name: Ondansetron hydrochloride
Brand Name: Zofran
Drug Class: Antiemetics, Selective 5-HT3 Antagonist
Used For: Prophylaxis and treatment of nausea and vomiting
Side Effects: See RxList.com

***Bri was frequently prescribed Zofran due to her nausea and vomiting. Bri could become very dehydrated from vomiting (even though she drank between 70-150 oz of water a day.) She'd end up in the hospital for hypokalemia and stay over-night for potassium infusions, being released once her potassium levels rose to low normal values. With the side effects of many of these medications being nausea and vomiting, a lot of her nausea could have been from the medications, although it also seems as if her disorder itself has nausea as a symptom. I have never seen nausea listed as a symptom of the disorder.

Generic Name: Oxybutynin
Brand Name: Ditropan
Drug Class: Antispasmotic, Urinary
Used For: Urinary Incontinence
Side Effects: Headaches, blurred vision, drowsiness, diarrhea, constipation
Serious Side Effects: See Rxlist.com

Generic Name: Paroxetine HCL
Brand Name: Paxil
Drug Class: Antidepressant, Selective Serotonin Reuptake Inhibitor (SSRI)

Used For: Depression, Obsessive-Compulsive Disorder (OCD), panic attacks, general anxiety, Post Traumatic Stress Disorder (PTSD)

Side Effects: Drowsiness, yawning, tiredness, anxiety, shaking, insomnia, nausea, headaches

Warning Box: Suicidal Ideation

Generic Name: Pazopanib

Brand Name: Votrient

Drug Class: Antineoplastics, VEGF Inhibitor, Antineoplastic Tyrosine Kinase Inhibitors

Used For: Treatment of Soft Tissue Sarcomas and Advanced Renal Cell Carcinoma

Side Effects: Hives, difficulty breathing, swelling of face, lips, tongue, or throat, unusual bleeding/bruising, slow healing of a wound, headache, confusion, seizure, nausea, see long list

Warning Box: see at Rxlist.com Serous Warnings

Generic Name: Prazosin Hydrochloride

Brand Name: Minipress

Drug Class: Alpha Adrenoreceptor Antagonists/Alpha Blocker (heart Medication)

Used For: This medication was used off label by Dr. PW for nightmares and it is listed for off label use

Side Effects: See RxList.com

*** We were really surprised at how effective Minipress was for reducing Bri's years of frequent horrific nightmares. She didn't have any side effects to it. She only had to take it for about a year and her nightmares were greatly reduced and have remained so.

Generic Name: Pregabalin

Brand Name: Lyrica

Drug Class: Fibromyalgia Agents, Anticonvulsants, Other

Used For: Nerve pain, neuropathic pain, fibromyalgia, partial-onset seizures when taken with other
            anti-seizure medications.

Side Effects: Ataxia, weight gain, tremor, swelling hands , feet, face, mouth, eyelids, tongue, sleepiness, dizziness, rash, hives, mania, panic attacks, insomnia, blurred vision

Warning Box: Suicidal Thoughts and Actions

***Bri quickly gained 10 pounds in 7 days and had swelling and blurred vision. Dr. RP immediately had her discontinue Lyrica.

Generic Name: Promethazine
Brand Name: Phenergan
Drug Class: Antiemetic Agent, 1st Generation Antihistamine
Used For: Treats allergic reactions, nausea, vomiting, motion sickness
Side Effects: Extreme drowsiness, seizures, uncontrolled muscle movements in the face, very stiff and rigid muscles, tremors, insomnia

Generic Name: Quetiapine Fumarate
Brand Name: Seroquel
Drug Class: Antipsychotic, Antimanic Agents, Atypical Antipsychotic Agent
Used For: Schizophrenia, Major Depressive Disorder, Bipolar Disorder
Side Effects: Uncontrolled facial muscles, rigid muscles, tremors, drowsiness, fast heartbeat,
Serious Side Effects: Tardive Dyskinesia (A movement disorder that can become permanent from taking psychoactive medications. Deep Brain Stimulation surgery is an option to treat it.)
Warning Box: Suicidal Ideation

Generic Name: Risperidone
Name Brand: Risperdal
Drug Class: Antipsychotics, S2nd Generation Antimanic Agent
Used For: Schizophrenia, Bipolar mania, Bipolar Disorder
Side Effects: Uncontrolled muscles in the face, rigid muscles, tremors\

Generic Name: Rizatriptan Benzoate
Brand Name: Maxalt
Drug Class: Serotonin 5-HT-Receptor Agonists, Antimigraine Agent
Used For: Migraines
Side Effects: Severe headache, nausea, muscle stiffness, twitching, slurred speech

Generic Name: Sumatriptan
Brand Name: Imitrex
Drug Class: Serotonin 5-HT-Receptor Agonists, Antimigraine Agents

Used For: Migraines
Side Effects: Seizure, irregular heartbeats, leg cramps, nausea, muscle stiffness, loss of coordination, slurred speech, poor balance, sudden severe headache, uneasy feeling
Warning Box: See list in RxList.com

Generic Name: Sumatriptan injectable
Brand Name: Sumavel Dosepro
Drug Class: Serotonin 5-HT-Receptor Agonists, Antimigraine Agents
Used For: Migraines
Side Effects: Heartbeat irregularities, fast heart rate, severe headache, anxiety, seizure, cramps in legs and feet,nausea
Serious Side Effects: Over active reflexes

Generic Name: Tizanidine
Brand Name: Zanaflex
Drug Class: Alpha 2 Adrenergic Agonist
Used For: Muscle spasticity
Side Effects: Fatigue, drowsiness, uncontrollable muscle movements
Serious Warnings: Liver toxicity, see list on RxList.com

***Bri still takes this medication at night and she seems to do well on it.

Generic name: Topirmate
Brand Name: Topomas
Drug Class: Anticonvulsant, Other, Antimigraine Agent
Used For: Seizures, migraines, and off label use for OCD
Side Effects: See list at RxList.com
(As a pharmacy tech, we were told the nickname of "Dopamax" because Topomax can interfere with cognitive functioning.)

***Off label use worked well to tamp down the OCD features of this disorder
***It was also used for decreasing the frequency of Bri's migraines and she took it for a year and it did indeed reduce the frequency of her migraines and she hasn't had to take it since then.

Generic Name: Trazodone Hydrochloride
Brand Name: Deseryl
Drug Class: Selective Serotonin Reuptake Inhibitor

Used For: Major Depressive Disorder
Side Effects: See list at RxList.com
Warning Box: Serious side effects and death. Suicidal Thoughts and Behaviors

***Bri was prescribed Trazodone at 15 years old for sleep, 50 mg at bedtime, but it never seemed to work, although she has remained on it for 16 years. She only slept 3-4 hours a night pre-surgery and sometimes she wouldn't sleep for up to 3 nights in a row. One time she didn't sleep for 6 nights in a row and had hallucinations. Since her DBS surgery, her neurologist increased her dosage to 100 to 150mg a night. She has found that the 150mg is too much and over time the 50mg seems to help her sleep along with the DBS surgery.

Generic Name: Venlafaxine HCL
Brand Name: Effexor
Drug Class: Antidepressant
Side Effects: Increased anxiety, increased panic attacks, increased depression and insomnia
Warning Box: Suicidal Ideation

Generic Name: Zonisamide
Brand Name: Zonegran
Drug Class: Anticonvulsant, Other
Used For: Treating partial seizures
Side Effects: Serious skin rash can cause death, problems with concentration and memory, thinking and speech, serious eye problems.
Serious Side Effects: See RxList.com
Warning Box: Suicidal Thoughts and Actions
***Dr. BA, Bri's DBS neuro, before surgery had her try Zonegran to see if it would alleviate her symptoms. After reviewing her medical history, along with all of the medications that she had tried over the years, told her that this was the last medication he would have her try. He did warn her that if she started having cognitive issues, to throw the medication out the window, far, far away! Within 2 weeks she was having issues so she quit taking the medication and it was on to surgery. No more trying to treat her Myoclonus Dystonia with medications only.

After reviewing this list of medications, I have several thoughts. My first thought is wow! All sorts of medications were tried and to no avail and with some serious side effects; including suicidal behaviors, rapid weight gain, and black out seizures. Her first black out seizure, Bri totaled her car and it could have been deadly! The second thought relates to how frightening it is to see how many medications, with their various side effects, and some serious, were used at the same time, sometimes up to seven medications at a time and started all at once! The third thought I have is just how many medications have Suicidal Ideation and Behaviors as a side effect. You might think that the pharmaceutical manufacturers are just "covering their asses" with this language, but Bri really did experience this serious side effect to several of the medications. It pays to be very vigilant when they list this side effect or have a Warning Box regarding serious side effects! The fourth take away I have is how many of the medications had side effects that were also symptoms of Myoclonus Dystonia and how they might have actually exacerbated Bri's symptoms.

The final thought I have relates to the idea that drinking alcohol, "If it helped," was possibly a safer approach to treating her Myoclonus Dystonia than taking the various cocktails of medications that she was prescribed. It seemed at the time that "taking" only one substance was the better option than taking the cocktails of the medications used to treat this disorder. Because her diagnosing specialist advised her to drink if it helped when the medications failed, as they so often do with this disorder, it seemed a safe option. Alcohol is known to be very effective in treating this disorder, also known as Alcohol Responsive Dystonia. It is shocking at how naïve I was at the time, and for many years later, about just how dangerous drinking alcohol is for an individual with this disorder.

Bri sees a pediatric neurologist/movement disorder specialist who specializes in Myoclonus Dystonia. He has shared his philosophy with us that he prefers to perform Deep Brain Stimulation surgery as soon as possible in children so that they don't have to experience the many medications and their side effects over the years. He says that many of the children, some very young, are put on psychoactive medications that do nothing to alleviate their symptoms and they cause so much trouble over time and aren't necessary. We experienced the prescribing of psychoactive medications when Bri was misdiagnosed with Bipolar I Disorder, the medications almost killed her so we agree with his early intervention idea. He also wants to intercede before a child figures out on their own that alcohol effectively reduces their symptoms but they end up with alcohol abuse issues that they have to deal with on top of everything else like Bri did. He is aware that specialists are still giving advice to "Drink if it helps" to individuals with Myoclonus Dystonia. I believe his youngest patient so far has been 7 years old and he is in the process of getting approval for a 5 year old with Myoclonus Dystonia to have DBS surgery. In the UK, a 2 year old has had a successful surgery recently.

I have also become suspicious that Bri has Multiple Drug Intolerance Syndrome because of her various reactions, and side effects, to multiple medications that aren't pharmacologically related. According to the American Academy of Allergy, Asthma, and Immunology, Multiple Drug Intolerance Syndrome is defined as: "Having greater than 3 or more unrelated drug intolerances or allergies." It also states that: "The more medications one is exposed to over time, the more likely an adverse drug reaction will occur." This certainly seems to be a possible explanation for all of Bri's reactions to her various medications, something to keep in mind.